DATE DUE

AUG 2 9 2002			

MICROLAPAROSCOPY

EDITED BY

OSCAR D. ALMEIDA, JR., M.D.

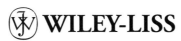

WILEY-LISS

A JOHN WILEY & SONS, INC., PUBLICATION

NEW YORK • CHICHESTER • WEINHEIM • BRISBANE • SINGAPORE • TORONTO

For ordering and customer service, call 1-800-CALL-WILEY.

Library of Congress Cataloging-in-Publication Data:
Microlaparoscopy/edited by Oscar D. Almeida, Jr.
    p.; cm.
  Includes bibliographical references and index.
  ISBN 0-471-34574-1 (cloth: alk. paper)
  1. Generative organs, Female--Endoscopic surgery, 2. Microsurgery, 3. Laparoscopic surgery. I. Almeida,
Oscar D.
  [DNLM: 1. Genital Diseases, Female--surgery, 2. Ambulatory Surgical Procedures--methods, 3. Micro-
surgery--methods, 4. Surgical procedures, Laparoscopic--methods. WP 660 M625 2000]
  RG104.7 M53 2000
  618'.0459--dc21   99-046509

Printed in the United States of America.

10 9 8 7 6 5 4 3 2 1

This book is dedicated to the memory of my father,
Oscar Almeida, Sr.

CONTENTS

FOREWORD

In the development of microlaparoscopic surgery under local anesthesia in an office setting, Oscar Almeida has become a respected leader. This concise and highly readable text is the first one to deal exclusively with this subject. In fulfilling his additional role as a superb teacher, Dr. Almeida continues to offer a thorough and well-designed two-day course in microlaparoscopy, which serves as a credentialing instrument (see Chapter 13).

Chapter 3 clearly outlines basic equipment and instrument needs. Analgesics, anesthetics, and safety precautions are addressed in Chapter 4. John Val-Gallas reveals his emphasis on compassionate patient-centered care in pre-op and post-op counseling in Chapter 5.

Important distinctions are made in Chapters 8 and 9 between operations appropriate for the office surgery and those of greater surgical complexity that most gynecologists prefer to schedule in the hospital operating room under general anesthesia.

Tubal sterilization operations are described in Chapter 8. In the same chapter Dr. Almeida discusses microlaparoscopic appendectomy under local anesthesia after pain mapping for chronic pelvic pain that reveals inordinate appendiceal tenderness. Microlaparoscopic ovarian drilling under local anesthesia for polycystic ovarian syndrome is fully described in Chapter 12.

Botros Rizk and Mostafa Abuzeid have demonstrated in Chapters 10 and 11 that microlaparoscopic procedures in infertility management and assisted reproductive technology can also be performed safely in the office under local anesthesia.

This persuasive and articulate book has succeeded in proving the important place of microlaparoscopy in modern gynecologic care and will serve as an authoritative reference as we enter the twenty-first century.

A. Jefferson Penfield, M.D., F.A.C.O.G.

PREFACE

Minimally invasive gynecologic surgery continues to revolutionize and redefine contemporary medicine. Advances in technique and instrumentation have led to this cutting-edge method known as microlaparoscopy. *Microlaparoscopy* is geared toward the gynecologist and general surgeon who will in the near future be forced to provide laparoscopic surgery in a more minimally invasive and cost-effective manner. The purpose of this book is to serve as an instructional tool to clinicians who are not yet performing microlaparoscopy and as a source of reference to those who are. It offers detailed guidance on all aspects of microlaparoscopy, including diagnostic and operative procedures under local anesthesia. The references have been carefully selected and purposefully limited. Reproductive endocrinologists will benefit from these techniques as the field of assisted reproductive technology (ART) continues to expand. Being the first textbook devoted in its entirety to microlaparoscopy, this book should serve as a foundation for future treatises.

The contributing authors bring a wealth of information to this book. John M. Val-Gallas, M.D., has been involved with our microlaparoscopy program since its inception. Botros Rizk, M.D., who trained under infertility pioneers Professor Robert Edwards and Dr. Patrick Steptoe brings his unique perspective on microlaparoscopy in the evaluation and treatment of infertility. Mostafa I. Abuzeid, M.D., shares his microlaparoscopic experience in ART from the work done at his center.

The reader will find many historic concepts revisited and miniaturized, which will broaden the knowledge of the laparoscopic surgeon. The use of these techniques will assist in the delivery of laparoscopic surgery in a minimally invasive manner. I would like to thank personally Mr. Shawn Morton of John Wiley & Sons, Inc. for his continued support during the writing of this textbook.

Oscar D. Almeida, Jr., M.D., F.A.C.O.G., F.A.C.S.

CONTRIBUTORS

MOSTAFA I. ABUZEID, M.D., F.A.C.O.G., F.R.C.O.G.
Associate Professor
Department of Obstetrics and Gynecology
Michigan State University College of Human Medicine
Flint, Michigan
Director, Division of Reproductive Endocrinology
Hurley Medical Center
Flint, Michigan

OSCAR D. ALMEIDA, JR., M.D., F.A.C.O.G., F.A.C.S.
Clinical Associate Professor
Department of Obstetrics and Gynecology
University of South Alabama College of Medicine
Mobile, Alabama
Chief, Division of Gynecology
U.S.A. Knollwood Park Hospital
Mobile, Alabama

BOTROS RIZK, M.D., M.A., M.R.C.O.G., F.R.C.S.(C.), H.C.L.D., F.A.C.O.G., F.A.C.S.
Associate Professor
Director, Division of Reproductive Endocrinology
Department of Obstetrics and Gynecology
University of South Alabama College of Medicine
Mobile, Alabama

JOHN M. VAL-GALLAS, M.D., F.A.C.O.G., F.A.C.S.
Private Practice
Mobile, Alabama

HISTORY OF MICROLAPAROSCOPY

OSCAR D. ALMEIDA, JR., M.D., F.A.C.O.G., F.A.C.S.

No chronicle of laparoscopy is complete without mention of the first recorded attempted visualization of the interior of a body cavity in 1805 by Bozzani of Frankfurt (1). Using a tool which he called a Lichtleiter and a candle as the light source, he visualized the urethra of a living person. His new innovation, however, was not met with praise. The medical faculty of Vienna investigated his visualization of hidden areas of the body, which was thought at that time to be unacceptable. He was scolded for his undue curiosity, and it was announced that his device was "a mere toy. "Investigations of this nature were discontinued until around 1880 when Nitze (2) developed the cystoscope.

Crude techniques and instrumentation at the turn of the twentieth century made laparoscopic evaluation cumbersome and challenging to the clinician. Primitive laparoscopes with inferior lighting and image transmission, poor anesthetic methods and untested laparoscopic techniques provided limited useful data. In 1901, Kelling (3) reported visualizing the stomach and esophagus of a dog using a Nitze cystoscope. During the same year, Ott (4) described the inspection of the abdominal cavity of a pregnant women using a head mirror and speculum inserted through a culdoscopic entry.

In 1910, Jacobaeus (5) of Stockholm coined the term laparoscopy and reported the first human laparoscopy using a Nitze cystoscope to inspect the peritoneal, pleural, and pericardial cavities. His technique did not involve creating a pneumoperitoneum before insertion of the trocar. Bernheim (6), an assistant surgeon at the Johns Hopkins University, performed the first laparoscopy in the United States, in 1911, using a half-inch diameter proctoscope through an epigastric incision.

Anesthetic methods for laparoscopy were inconsistent. In 1925, Short (7) described his technique for the use of local anesthesia in laparoscopic

Microlaparoscopy, Edited by Oscar D. Almeida Jr.
ISBN 0-471-34574-1   Copyright © 2000 by Wiley-Liss, Inc.

surgery. Fervers (8) was the first to report on operative laparoscopy when he lysed adhesions and performed several intra-abdominal biopsies. Veress (9) of Hungary introduced a needle for creating a pneumothorax in the management of tuberculosis during an era of limited pharmacologic means. Although its initial purpose was unsuccessful, this needle is commonly used today for creating a pneumoperitoneum in laparoscopic surgery. Decker and Cherry (10) reported using the knee-chest position and creating a pneumoperitoneum through the cul-de-sac under local anesthesia. They called this procedure *culdoscopy* and believed that it was less painful than laparoscopy and produced complete visualization of the pelvic structures.

Palmer of France in the 1940s and Steptoe of England in the 1960s pioneered laparoscopic techniques for gynecology and reproductive medicine. Owing to his extensive contributions in this field, Palmer (11) is considered to be the father of contemporary gynecologic laparoscopy. Using the Trendelenburg position for improved visualization of the pelvic cavity, he performed *peritoneoscopy* in his private clinic under general anesthesia. Palmer developed several surgical instruments for his procedures and underscored the importance of monitoring intra-abdominal pressures during laparoscopy. Palmer and his associate Klein (12) were the first to report the retrieval of human oocytes through the laparoscope in 1961.

In 1967, Steptoe (13) published the first book in the English language on laparoscopy. His book *Laparoscopy in Gynecology* contained the first description of laparoscopic sterilization using monopolar cautery and detailed many other laparoscopic procedures, such as ovarian biopsies, lysis of adhesions, uterine suspension, and appendectomy. In 1978, he and his colleague Edwards reported in *The Lancet* their landmark paper detailing the first successful human *in vitro* conception and birth of baby Louise Brown. To further the exchange of knowledge in the field of laparoscopy, Phillips (15) founded the American Association of Gynecologic Laparoscopists in 1971.

Wheeles (16) in 1972 reported 3600 cases of outpatient sterilization using local anesthesia and popularized the concept of outpatient surgery. In 1973, Hulka and colleagues (17) developed a spring-loaded clip; and in 1974 Yoon et al. (18) introduced a Falope ring technique for laparoscopic tubal sterilization. In 1972, Penfield (19) introduced technical modifications in outpatient laparoscopy under local anesthesia to improve safety, economy, and patient acceptability. He reported 22 years of experience in 1995 of more than 2450 laparoscopic cases done under local anesthesia in the office or free-standing clinic. During the 1970s, Semm (20) developed new techniques with fiber optics for operative laparoscopy and introduced the automatic CO_2 insufflator. Also during this period, Kleppinger (21), Corson and co-workers (22), Rioux and co-workers (23) developed the bipolar method of electrosurgery for tubal sterilization. In response to the potential risk of injury resulting from blind trocar or Veress needle insertion, Hasson (24) developed a cannula for open laparoscopy.

The 1980s provided generalized acceptance of laparoscopy by gynecologists, both diagnostic and operative, using the 10- and 12-mm rod lens laparoscopes. During this decade, laparoscopy became the procedure of choice for removal of ectopic pregnancies, interval sterilization, and infertility evaluations. As part of the obstetrics and gynecology training, laparoscopy was introduced into the curriculum for residency programs. Many procedures previously done only via laparotomy were now being attempted with laparoscopy. Macrolaparoscopy flourished with improved laparoscopes, lasers, and other instrumentation (e.g., cautery scissors and Endoloop suturing).

Miniaturization of laparoscopes made a brief appearance in 1976 when Dingfelder and Brenner (25) reported using the 1.7- and 2.2-mm diameter rod lens "needlescopes" for tubal sterilization and diagnostic procedures. Unfortunately, poor resolution severely limited their usefulness, and small laparoscopes remained dormant for over a decade. In 1991, Dorsey and Tabb (26) described using a 3-mm laparoscope and 3-mm instrumentation, including grasping forceps, biopsy forceps, and scissors under general anesthesia in a procedure that they called *mini-laparoscopy*. Childers and his colleagues (27) first reported the usefulness of performing biopsies under local anesthesia in the office setting using small-diameter laparoscopes in patients with intra-abdominal malignancies.

Risquez and co-workers (28) in 1993 reported doing *microlaparoscopy* under local anesthesia with conscious sedation. They encountered problems with picture resolution in the microlaparoscopes. As technology improved, they suggested replacing *macro*laparoscopy with the more minimally invasive technique of *micro*laparoscopy. Steege (29) illustrated the benefits of repeated clinic laparoscopy for the treatment of pelvic adhesions. Bauer and co-workers (30) and Feste (31) reported the use of optical catheters for diagnostic office laparoscopy. Palter and Olive (32) described the concept of *conscious pain mapping* for the evaluation of women with chronic pelvic pain. Demco (33) presented a similar concept, which he called *patient assisted laparoscopy*.

With the newly introduced concept of conscious pain mapping, Almeida et al. (34) developed a classification for conscious pain mapping and described the importance of the appendix as an etiology of chronic pelvic pain using the technique of microlaparoscopic conscious pain mapping. Later, Almeida and co-workers (36) pioneered a protocol for conscious sedation useful for both diagnostic and operative microlaparoscopic procedures, including electrosurgery to fulgurate endometriosis, primary lysis of adhesions, and laparoscopic uterosacral nerve ablation (LUNA). In 1998, Almeida's group (37) opened the field of operative microlaparoscopy under local anesthesia when they reported the first microlaparoscopic appendectomies for the treatment of chronic pelvic pain; the first microlaparoscopic ovarian drilling for the surgical treatment of polycystic ovary syndrome was reported the same year (38). These advances have unlocked the door for additional operative microlaparoscopic procedures currently under research protocols.

The twentieth century brought many innovations for the evaluation and treatment of gynecologic patients with chronic pelvic pain, infertility, and undesired fertility. Myriad techniques and instrumentation changes mark the advances that have led to microlaparoscopy today as we enter the new millennium. With the introduction of microlaparoscopy, a new era in gynecologic laparoscopic surgery continues to evolve (39). Operative microlaparoscopy under local anesthesia is now possible for the treatment of endometriosis, primary lysis of adhesions, and assisted reproductive technology (ART) in selected patients. These minimally invasive techniques produce less surgical trauma, are less expensive to perform, and allow the patient to return back to her normal routine more quickly than more traditional procedures. Minimally invasive microlaparoscopic surgery is the way of the future.

REFERENCES

1. Belt AE, Charnock DA. The history of the cystoscope. In Cabol H, ed., Modern urology. Philadelphia: Lea & Febiger, 1936:15–50.

2. Nitze M. Uber eine neue Beleuchtungsmethode der Hohlen des menschlichen Korpers. Wien Med Presse 20:851–858, 1879.

3. Kelling G. Uber Oesophagoskopie, Gastroskopie und Koelioskopie. Munch Med Wochenschr 49(1): 21–24, 1902.

4. Ott DO. Ventroscopic illumination of the abdominal cavity in pregnancy. Zh Akusher Zhensk Boleznei 15:7–8, 1901.

5. Jacobaeus HC. Uber die Moglichkeit die Zystoskopie bei Untersuchung seroser Hohlungen anzuwenden. Munch Med Wochenschr 57:2090–2092, 1910.

6. Bernheim BM. Organoscopy: cystoscopy of the abdominal cavity. Ann Surg 53:764–767, 1911.

7. Short AR. The uses of coelioscopy. Br Med J 222:254–255, 1925.

8. Fervers C. Die Laparoskopie mit dem cystoskop: ein beitrag zur vereinfachung der technik und zur endoskopischen Strangdurtrennung in der Bauchhohle. Med Klin 29:1042–1045, 1933.

9. Veress J. Neues instrument zur Ausfuhrung von Brust-oder Bauchpumptionen und Pneumothorax behanddlung. Dtsch Med Wochenschr 64:1480, 1938.

10. Decker A, Cherry T. Culdoscopy: a new method in diagnosis of pelvic disease—preliminary report. Am J Surg 64:40–44, 1944.

11. Palmer R. Instrumentation et technique de la coelioscopie gynecologique. Gynecol Obstet 46:420–431, 1947.

12. Klein R, Palmer R. Technique de preelevement des ovules humaines par ponction folliculaire sans coelioscopie. C R Soc Biol (Paris) 155:1918–1921, 1961.

13. Steptoe PC. Laparoscopy in gynecology. Edinburgh: Livingston, 1967.

14. Steptoe PC, Edwards RG. Birth after the reimplantation of a human embryo. Lancet 366:2–5, 1978.

15. Phillips JM. Changes. J Am Assoc Gynecol Laparosc 4:153–156, 1997.

16. Wheeles CR Jr. Outpatient laparoscopic sterilization under local anesthesia. Obstet Gynecol 39:767–770, 1972.

17. Hulka JF, Fishburne JI, Mercer JP, et al. Laparoscopic sterilization with a spring clip: a report of the first fifty cases. Am J Obstet Gynecol 116:715–718, 1973.

18. Yoon IB, Wheeless CR Jr, King TM. A preliminary report on a new laparoscopic sterilization approach: the silicone rubber band technique. Am J Obstet Gynecol 120:132–136, 1974.

19. Penfield AJ. Twenty-two years of office and outpatient laparoscopy: current techniques and why I chose them. J Am Assoc Gynecol Laparosc 2:365–368, 1995.

20. Semm K. Atlas of gynecologic laparoscopy and hysteroscopy. Philadelphia: Saunders, 1977.

21. Kleppinger RK. Female outpatient sterilization using bipolar coagulation. Bull Post-Grad Committee Med, (U Sydney), Nov:144–154, 1977.

22. Corson SL, Patrick H, Hamilton T, Bolognese RJ. Electrical consideration of laparoscopic sterilization. J Reprod Med 11:159–164, 1973.

23. Rioux J, Cloutier D. Bipolar cautery for sterilization by laparoscopy. J Reprod Med 13: 6–10, 1974.

24. Hasson HM. Open laparoscopy: a report of 150 cases. J Reprod Med 12:234–238, 1974.

25. Dingfelder JR, Brenner WE. The needlescope and other small diameter laparoscopes for sterilization and diagnostic procedures. Int J Gynaecol Obstet 14:53–58, 1976.

26. Dorsey JH, Tabb CR. Mini-laparoscopy and fiber-optic lasers. Obstet Gynecol Clin N Am 18:613–617, 1991.

27. Childers JM, Hatch KD, Surwit EA. Office laparoscopy and biopsy for evaluation of patients with intraperitoneal carcinomatosis using a new optical catheter. 47:337–342, 1992.

28. Risquez F, Pennehouat G, Fernandez R, et al. Microlaparoscopy: a preliminary report. Hum Repro 8:1701–1702, 1993.

29. Steege J. Repeated clinic laparoscopy for the treatment of pelvic adhesions: A pilot study. Obstet Gynecol 83:276–279, 1994.

30. Bauer O, Devroey P, Wisanto A, et al. Small diameter laparoscopy using a microlaparoscope. Hum Repro 8:1461–1464, 1993.

31. Feste J. Use of optical catheters for diagnostic office laparoscopy. J Reprod Med 41:307–312, 1996.

32. Palter SF, Olive DL. Office microlaparoscopy under local anesthesia for chronic pelvic pain. J Am Assoc Gynecol Laparosc 3:359–364, 1996.

33. Demco LA. Patient-assisted laparoscopy. J Am Assoc Gynecol laparosc S8, 1996.

34. Almeida OD Jr, Val-Gallas JM, Rizk B. A novel classification for conscious pain mapping. Egy J Fertil Steril 1:53–58, 1997.

35. Almeida OD Jr, Val-Gallas JM. Conscious pain mapping. J Am Assoc Gynecol Laparosc 4:587–590, 1997.

36. Almeida OD Jr, Val-Gallas JM, Browning JL. A protocol for conscious sedation in microlaparoscopy. J Am Assoc Gynecol Laparosc 4:591–594, 1997.

37. Almeida OD Jr, Val-Gallas JM, Rizk B. Appendectomy under local anaesthesia following conscious pain mapping with microlaparoscopy. Hum Reprod 13:588–590, 1998.

38. Almeida OD Jr, Val-Gallas JM. Microlaparoscopic ovarian drilling under local anesthesia. Middle East Fertil Soc J 3:189–191, 1998.

39. Almeida OD Jr, Rizk B. Microlaparoscopy: its evolution, present and future. Middle East Fertil Soc J 3:1–2, 1998.

INFORMED CONSENT

OSCAR D. ALMEIDA, JR., M.D., F.A.C.O.G., F.A.C.S.

Helping our patients make rational decisions before surgery is an important part of the practice of medicine (1). Ethical and legal obligations underscore the necessity to provide and obtain adequate informed consent. Proper informed consent includes the understanding by the patient of relevant factors of the proposed surgical procedure. This permission, approval, or assent given to a surgeon implies that adequate discussion has taken place between the surgeon and patient regarding the disorder to be treated; proposed surgical procedure; risks; likelihood of success with the procedure; and alternate forms of therapy, including medical therapy, laparotomy and no treatment at all. No guarantee of success or false assurance that the procedure lacks risk should be conveyed to the patient. This interactive partnership involving the surgeon and patient must be realized before any elective surgical procedure, such as microlaparoscopy. Exceptions to informed consent include life-threatening emergencies in the unconscious patient and if the risk of failure to treat are higher than the risks of treatment.

HISTORICAL PERSPECTIVES

Historically, the roots of informed consent were established under English common law by the case *Slater vs. Baker & Stapleton* (2) heard by the King's Bench in 1767 in which the plaintiff alleged negligence and lack of informed consent for a surgical procedure. This concept was continued in 1905 in *Mohr vs. Williams* (3). In *Mohr*, a surgeon was given consent to operate on a patient's right ear. Finding the left ear in need of surgical care, the surgeon operated on the left ear with success. He did not, however, obtain informed consent for the additional procedure. Performing the unauthorized procedure was held to be assault and battery.

Microlaparoscopy, Edited by Oscar D. Almeida, Jr.
ISBN 0-471-34574-1   Copyright © 2000 by Wiley-Liss, Inc.

Contemporary American law was first established in 1914 in the case of *Schloendorf vs. Society of New York Hospital* (4). Judge B. Cardozo ruled that "every human being of adult years and sound mind has a right to determine what shall be done with their own body; and a surgeon who performs an operation without his patient's consent, commits an assault for which he is liable for damages." The term *informed consent* was first used in 1957 in the California case *Salgo vs. Leland Stanford Jr* (5). Before 1972, the medical community determined what constituted adequate informed consent (6, 7). In 1972 the case of *Canterbury vs. Spence* withdrew the right to determine what must be disclosed to patients by the medical profession (8). The Canterbury court affirmed that "every human being of adult years and sound mind has a right to determine what shall be done with their own body." The American Medical Association (AMA) has stated, "The patient's right of self-determination can be effectively exercised only if the patient possesses enough information to enable an intelligent choice" (9).

INFORMED CONSENT IN MICROLAPAROSCOPY

Informed consent must cover all aspects of the surgical procedure in microlaparoscopy. This includes the procedure itself and anesthesia/analgesia. Because microlaparoscopic procedures are usually elective in nature, these dialogues should be undertaken in the physicians office during the preoperative consultation. In addition to open discussions with the patient and family, newsletters, videos, and brochures may assist in providing proper patient information. Informed consent cannot be legally obtained from a patient who is under the influence of medications or other factors that might interfere with her rational judgment.

In some patients with chronic pelvic pain and/or infertility, a precise diagnosis cannot be made preoperatively. A discussion of the possible expected surgical findings—such as endometriosis, adhesions, and tubal occlusion—in addition to which procedures will be performed at the time of surgery to address these findings should be undertaken. Diagnostic microlaparoscopy is frequently followed by operative microlaparoscopy. Therefore, conversations should include possible further procedures that may be necessary to correct the problem(s) in question. For example, extensive surgery including laparotomy, hysterectomy, and/or salpingo-oophorectomy may be required in cases of severe endometriosis.

If the microlaparoscopic procedure is to be conducted in an office laparoscopy suite, it may be appropriate to discuss with the patient the adequacy of the surgical facility. Knowing that such a facility has all appropriately trained personnel and emergency equipment will help decrease the patient's anxiety during surgery. The types of anesthesia/analgesia and what the patient should expect during and after the operation should be presented. For example, an awake procedure done under local anesthesia with conscious sedation requires extensive patient participation; therefore, such patients should receive a more detailed account of what to expect.

The possibility of a laparotomy due to hemorrhage, bowel or bladder perforation, or hypovolemic shock should be discussed. Other complications including infection, incisional hernia, and even death must be stated. Patient complaints following laparoscopic surgery vary with the type of procedure done (10). Excessive informed consent, however, may lead to unnecessary fears, confusion, and anxiety for the patient and family (11). Nevertheless, before a surgical procedure, informed written consent must be obtained (Fig. 2.1).

Consent Form For Microlaparoscopy

Patient's Name_____ Date_____

I authorize and direct_____M.D. and his assistant(s) of his choice to medically/surgically treat the condition(s) considered to be present in my case.

The microlaparoscope is a small telescope-like instrument which is inserted through a small incision in the umbilicus. The abdominal cavity is distended with a gas medium (usually carbon dioxide) as an aid to better visualize the contents of the pelvic and abdominal cavities with the microlaparoscope. One or more additional small incisions may be required to insert other instruments to perform the surgical procedure. The procedure may be done under local anesthesia with conscious sedation or general anesthesia.

Video and/or still pictures may be taken during the surgical procedure. These videos and/or still pictures are used to illustrate the surgical findings to the patient and may be used to teach other doctors and/or patients. I am aware that visiting surgeons may observe my microlaparoscopic procedure.

Although complications from microlaparoscopy are very rare, they can occur. These may include,but not limited to, hemorrhage, hematoma, hypovolemic shock, injury to the urinary or gastrointestinal tract, hernia or infection. Some of these complications may require emergency major abdominal/pelvic surgery. The risks of catastrophic complications such as death, paralysis, colostomy or requiring a hysterectomy are rare.

I am aware that in surgical procedures, other unexpected risks or complications not discussed may occur. I also understand that during the course of the proposed surgical procedure(s) unforseen conditions may be revealed requiring the performance of additional procedures, and I authorize such procedures to be performed. I further acknowledge that no guarantees or promises have been made to me concerning the results of any procedure or treatment.

My signature below acknowledges that I have read the contents of this consent form, understand and agree with the foregoing, that the proposed surgical procedure(s) have been satisfactorily explained to me including possible risks and alternative treatment plans. I hereby give my informed, voluntary authorization and consent.

DO NOT SIGN THIS FORM UNLESS YOU HAVE READ IT, UNDERSTAND IT AND AGREE WITH WHAT IT SAYS.

Signature:
Date:
Witness:
Date:

FIGURE 2.1. Sample consent form.

REFERENCES

1. Redelmeir DA, Rozin P, Kahneman D. Understanding patients' decisions. JAMA 270:72–76, 1993.

2. *Baker vs. Stapleton*, 2 Wils. K.B.359, 95 Eng. Rep. 860, 1767.

3. *Mohr vs. Williams*, 95 Minn. 261, 104 N.W. 12 , 1905.

4. *Schloendorf vs. Society of New York Hospital*, 105 NE 92, 1914.

5. *Salgo vs. Leland Stanford Jr. and the University Board of Trustees*, 154 Cal. App. 2d 560, 317 P.2d 670, 1957.

6. *Danielson vs. Roche*, 109 Cal. App.2d 832, 835, 241 P.2d 1028, 1030, 1952.

7. *Engelking vs. Carlson*, 13 Cal. 2d 216, 88 P.2d 695, 1939.

8. *Canterbury vs. Spence*, 464 F.2d 772-789 (D.C. Cir.), 1972.

9. American Medical Association's statement on informed consent. Mutual Assurance of Alabama Malpractice Seminar, Mobile, Alabama, 1999.

10. Azziz R, Steinkampf MP, Murphy A. Postoperative recuperation: relation to the extent of endoscopic surgery. Fertil Steril 51:1061–1064, 1989.

11. Stenchever MA. Too much informed consent? Obstet Gynecol 77:631, 1991.

MICROLAPAROSCOPIC EQUIPMENT

OSCAR D. ALMEIDA, JR., M.D., F.A.C.O.G., F.A.C.S.

MICROLAPAROSCOPES

The advances in microlaparoscopy celebrated today have resulted from the recent progress made in fiberoptic technology. Microlaparoscopy refers to the use of small-diameter laparoscopes ($<$ 2-mm in diameter) that are made of microfiber optics bundles measured in micrometers (1). Minilaparoscopy can be confused with minilaparotomy; it refers to small-diameter rod lens endoscopes, such as the needlescope (1).

Small endoscopes have been available for many years. Their use has been cataloged in otolaryngology, urology, and orthopedics. The challenge with developing today's microlaparoscopes was in creating a small laparoscope that illuminated enough light to enable the surgeon to see large, dark areas, such as the pelvic and abdominal cavities. Besides illumination problems, resolution (the laparoscopes' ability to detect a small object at a given distance, i.e., a spot of endometriosis) and durability presented difficulties.

Rod lenses as microlaparoscopes were not durable. The early rod lens needlescopes of the 1970s provided poor-quality visualization of the pelvic and abdominal cavities. Light-condensing technology was difficult to use with the rod lens. When the endoscope was bent, the lens would break, resulting in loss of image. These microlaparoscopes were expensive to repair and/or replace.

Fiberoptic lens endoscopes were primarily used for bronchoscopes and colonoscopes. They were typically dark, and each individual image fiber or pixel was independent of other fibers. The problem was that when a fiber burned out, a dark spot would appear on the screen, limiting the visual field.

The current 2-mm microlaparoscopes began to be developed around 1993. These were improved by adding more pixels to each microlaparo-

Microlaparoscopy, Edited by Oscar D. Almeida, Jr.
ISBN 0-471-34574-1   Copyright © 2000 by Wiley-Liss, Inc.

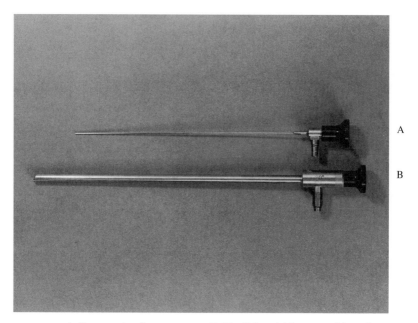

FIGURE 3.1. **A**, 2-mm microlaparoscope. **B**, Traditional 10-mm rod lens laparoscope.

scope (5,000 to 10,000 per scope). The illumination and resolution, however, remained poor. The breakthrough came with the introduction of *diffused image bundle* technology. It began with 15,000 pixels per microlaparoscope. Improved resolution and increased light-condensing technology were achieved. The first-generation 2-mm microlaparoscopes had 30,000 pixels. This enabled surgeons to perform both diagnostic and operative microlaparoscopy. The current second-generation gold series 2-mm microlaparoscopes (Minisite; U.S. Surgical Corp., Norwalk, CT) have a 50,000-fiber image bundle that produces enhanced resolution and a 75° field of view, comparable to a standard 10-mm rod lens laparoscope (Fig. 3.1). These microlaparoscopes can be bent and are more durable during handling and cleaning, which reduces the cost of repair and replacement.

CAMERAS AND ACCESSORY EQUIPMENT

There are many excellent laparoscopic cameras available commercially. Features that enhance the image detail and magnify the field of view on the television screen are particularly useful for microlaparoscopy. The Endovision Telecam SL camera (Karl Storz Endoscopy, Culver City, CA) has a parafocal zoom lensing system, which alleviates the need to refocus when magnifying the image (Fig. 3.2). Supplemental accessories, such as a camera box, light source, and cord, should be checked for compatibility with any particular camera system. Interchangeability of equipment from different

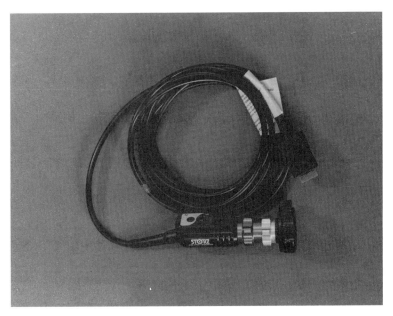

FIGURE 3.2. Camera used in microlaparoscopy.

manufacturers must be contemplated. An automatic insufflator for the pneumoperitoneum is standard equipment for any laparoscopic procedure.

MICROINSTRUMENTATION

Whether to employ single-use or reusable instrumentation in microlaparoscopy is a matter of personal preference, although the latter is more cost-effective. A full complement of 2-mm instruments are available for both diagnostic and operative microlaparoscopy.

TROCARS

Single-use 2-mm trocars that interlock with a Veress needle function well as primary trocars and avoid the need for two separate umbilical instrument insertions (Fig. 3.3, **A**). Once the pneumoperitoneum is created, the Veress needle is removed, leaving the trocar in place. This technology is helpful, because it saves a step and, in cases of suspected bowel perforation, the microlaparoscope can be readily inserted providing an instant diagnosis (2). These 2-mm cannulas have an insufflation port. The disposable Veress needle is beneficial because after repeated use, the tip of the nondisposable variety becomes dull. The reusable 2-mm trocars function well as secondary trocars and are very cost-effective (Fig. 3.3, **B**).

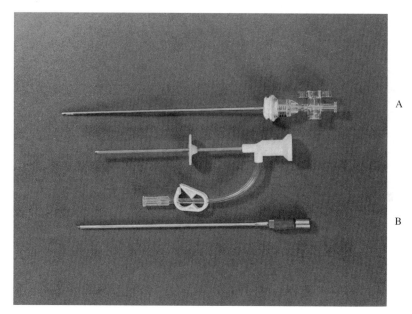

FIGURE 3.3. **A,** Single-use interlocking 2-mm trocar and Veress needle. **B,** Reusable 2-mm trocar.

PROBES

The 2-mm probe is useful for diagnostic and operative microlaparoscopy (Fig. 3.4, **A**). Its gradations, measured in centimeters, are helpful for measuring tubal length during evaluations for potential tubal anastomosis. We use this instrument to probe tissues, structures, and lesions during conscious pain mapping. It is effective for lysis of adhesions and other operative procedures by immobilization of structures.

IRRIGATION/ASPIRATION CANNULAS

The irrigation/aspiration cannula serves many functions (Fig. 3.4, **B**). For operative procedures, such as electrosurgery for the fulguration of endometiosis or lysis of adhesions, this cannula can provide a good stream of irrigation fluid or local anesthetic from an attached 20 ml syringe. Conversely, it works well to aspirate fluids.

INJECTION/ASPIRATION NEEDLE CANNULAS

The injection needle cannula is useful for cases requiring the injection of local anesthesia, such as when adequate analgesia is not achieved solely by

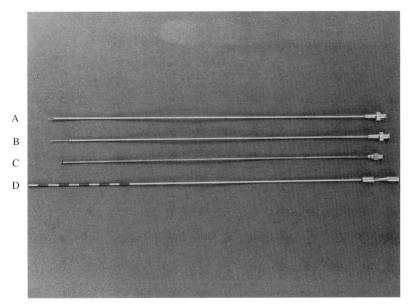

FIGURE 3.4. **A**, Large-bore aspiration needle cannula. **B**, A 23-gauge injection needle cannula. **C**, Irrigation/aspiration cannula. **D**, Blunt probe with centimeter markings.

the application of local anesthesia to the uterosacral ligament during a LUNA procedure (Fig. 3.4, **C**). A 23-gauge needle is used. The larger-bore aspiration needle cannula is used primarily for aspirating simple ovarian cysts (Fig. 3.4, **D**).

FORCEPS

Grasping forceps with serrated jaws and atraumatic grasping forceps are available in a 2-mm size (Fig. 3.5, **A,B**). The serrated jaws work well for grasping the appendix, whereas the atraumatic forceps are used for the more delicate structures, such as the ovaries and fallopian tubes. Biopsy forceps are used for sampling suspected endometrial implants or lesions on the ovaries or peritoneum seen during microlaparoscopy (Fig. 3.5, **C**).

SCISSORS

Reusable 2-mm noncautery scissors are effective for lysis of filmy (nonvascular) adhesions, dividing tissue coagulated with the bipolar forceps, and cutting Endoloop suture (Fig. 3.5, **D**). These scissors are available only in the straight-tip variety to fit through the small trocars. Monopolar 2-mm

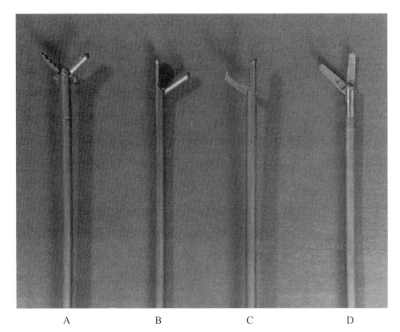

FIGURE 3.5. **A**, Serrated jaws of grasping forceps. **B**, Atraumatic jaws of grasping forceps for delicate work. **C**, Biopsy forceps. **D**, Straight-tip noncautery microlaparoscopic scissors.

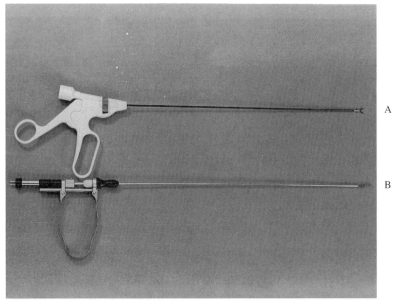

FIGURE 3.6. **A**, Monopolar cautery scissors. **B**, Bipolar forceps.

cautery scissors are available (Fig. 3.6, **A**), which are used for hemostasis, to fulgurate endometriosis implants, lyse adhesions, and perform LUNA.

BIPOLAR FORCEPS

The 2-mm bipolar forceps are a recent addition to the available microinstrumentation (Fig. 3.6, **B**). These are used primarily for hemostasis but work well for the bipolar coagulation method of tubal sterilization.

ENDOLOOPS

Endoloop suture is available in a 0 plain gut absorbable suture with a disposable 2-mm suture introducer (Fig. 3.7). It is useful for hemostasis as well as for tubal sterilization.

ACCESSORY EQUIPMENT

Uterine manipulators are used for uterine elevation or chromotubation. A HUME is used for chromotubation to evaluate tubal patency (Fig. 3.8, **A**). A Hulka tenaculum-sound is used for patients who have had a previous tubal sterilization procedure or when reproduction is not an issue (Fig. 3.8, **B**). A single-toothed tenaculum is used to grasp and stabilize the cervix (Fig. 3.8, **C**). A set of three reusable cervical dilators made of Teflon that can

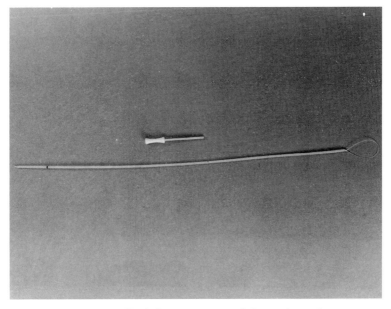

FIGURE 3.7. Endoloop suture and 2-mm introducer.

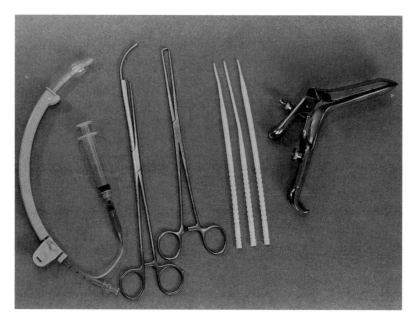

FIGURE 3.8. Accessory equipment for microlaparoscopy.

withstand autoclaving is invaluable (Fig. 3.8, **D**). The set includes a cervical os locator, a cervical canal finder, and a fundus dilator to open the internal cervical os. Finally, the introduction of these vaginal instruments are facilitated with the use of a side-open Graves speculum (Fig. 3.8, **E**).

REFERENCES

1. Risquez F. Microlaparoscopy: indications and applications. In Kempers RD, Cohen J, Haney AF, Younger JB, eds., Fertility and reproductive medicine. Amsterdam: Elsevier Science 1998:71–72.
2. Almeida OD Jr, Val-Gallas JM. Small trocar perforation of the small bowel: a case report. J Soc Laparoendosc Surg. 2:289–290, 1998.

ANESTHESIA/ANALGESIA

OSCAR D. ALMEIDA, JR., M.D., F.A.C.O.G., F.A.C.S. and
JOHN M. VAL-GALLAS, M.D., F.A.C.O.G., F.A.C.S.

Microlaparoscopy provides an excellent opportunity for a varied approach with anesthetic technique. General anesthesia is appropriate in certain situations, especially lengthy, complex procedures. General anesthesia, however, has been associated with most of the operative morbidity and mortality that occur with laparoscopy (1). Therefore, strong consideration should be given to the feasibility of performing microlaparoscopic procedures under local anesthesia with conscious sedation whenever possible.

Why use local anesthesia for microlaparoscopic surgeries? It has been well established that intubation, general anesthesia, and mechanical ventilation are not required for safe and effective microlaparoscopy (2). Postoperative complaints of sore throat, headaches, nausea, and vomiting noted after general anesthesia are usually not seen with procedures done under local anesthesia. In addition, the postoperative recovery period is shorter when local instead of general anesthesia is used. From an economic standpoint, general anesthesia is far more costly to the patient and insurance carrier in terms of dollars than local anesthesia with conscious sedation.

Why do a conscious microlaparoscopic procedure? First of all, the procedures are more minimally invasive than those performed under general anesthesia. Moreover, the conscious patient is helpful in making the diagnosis, especially in cases of chronic pelvic pain. In reviewing the protocols in the literature as well as feedback obtained from physicians, we have observed that there is a great misunderstanding between *conscious sedation* and *unconscious sedation*. Many clinicians are incorrectly labeling conscious sedation with what is truly unconscious sedation. Table 4.1 summarizes the differences between these two distinctly different levels of sedation.

Microlaparoscopy, Edited by Oscar D. Almeida, Jr.
ISBN 0-471-34574-1   Copyright © 2000 by Wiley-Liss, Inc.

TABLE 4-1. CONSCIOUS SEDATION VS. UNCONCIOUS SEDATION

Conscious Sedation

- A medically controlled state of depressed consciousness
- Allows the patient's protective reflexes to be maintained
- Retains the patient's ability to maintain a patent airway independently and continuously
- Permits appropriate patient response to questioning

Unconscious Sedation

- A medically controlled state of unconsciousness from which the patient is not easily aroused
- Partial or complete loss of the patient's protective reflexes
- Inability to maintain a patent airway independently
- Inability to repond purposefully

Safety presents a critical issue that must be addressed, especially if the surgical procedures are performed in an office-based, free-standing facility and the conscious sedation is administered by nonanesthesiologists. The physicians and registered nurse must be advanced cardiac life support (ACLS) certified to be able to address emergencies. The American Society of Anesthesiologists (ASA) (3) has published comprehensive guidelines for sedation and analgesia. These guidelines are summarized in Table 4.2.

The administration of drugs should be based on the patient's weight and doses titrated in a methodical way to ensure patient safety and a satisfactory level of sedation and analgesia. Outpatient anesthesia/analgesia for conscious microlaparoscopic procedures begins with patient selection. A thorough preanesthetic patient assessment is the single most important aspect for reducing the operative complication rate. This includes, but is not limited to, historical and current information regarding the patient's cardiovascular, respiratory, hepatic, renal, and cerebral function. Current medications, past surgical and anesthetic history, drug allergies, and review of systems. This is followed by a complete physical examination and

TABLE 4.2. SAFETY GUIDELINES FOR NONANESTHESIOLOGISTS

- Monitoring of respiratory rate and ventilatory function
- Use of a pulseoximeter
- Blood pressure monitoring
- Continuous electrocardiogram
- Continuous intravenous access
- Emergency and resuscitative equipment and drugs, including a defibrillator, and crashcart containing emergency drugs and reversal agents

laboratory testing. A battery of tests, including CBC, electrolytes, liver pro-file, urinalysis, HCG, EKG, and chest x-ray are done preoperatively. If the procedures are to be performed in an office laparoscopy suite where the conscious sedation is administered by nonanesthesiologists, then the patient's preoperative evaluation should place her at no higher than an (ASA) level 2 classification.

There is a multitude of pharmacologic agents that can be used in micro-laparoscopic procedures done under local anesthesia with conscious seda-tion. Some properties of analgesics and anxiolytics offer advantages within the group of choices. Ideally, an *analgesic agent* would have potent analgesic activity, minimal respiratory depression, little or no nausea associated with its use, no histamine release, and a short duration of action as well as evoke minimal euphoric or dysphoric response, and be easily reversed. The ideal *anxiolytic agent* would have potent anxiolytic properties, minimal respira-tory depression, and a short half-life as well as evoke minimal sedation and be reversible. Obviously, no currently available drug exhibits all the afore-mentioned properties. We employ and recommend those that in our experi-ence appear to come the closest.

ANALGESIC AGENTS

FENTANYL CITRATE

Fentanyl citrate is our narcotic analgesic of choice. It is a synthetic opioid compound with even greater potency than morphine. Advantages include a rapid onset of action and short period of bioavailability, low frequency of side effects, and short recovery period. Unlike morphine, histamine release is rarely a problem with fentanyl. Disadvantages of fentanyl include an oc-casional late respiratory depression and bradycardia, especially if large doses are administered quickly over a short period of time. Naloxone hy-drochloride is the reversal agent for fentanyl; however, because its half-life is short, more than one dose may be necessary.

MORPHINE

Morphine is still the standard against which other narcotics are compared for their analgesic properties. It does not affect cardiac contractility, although it does produce venous dilatation and mild lowering of blood pressure. The major disadvantages of morphine include histamine release, respiratory depression, and sedation. The latter is a drawback for conscious procedures, such as conscious pain mapping. Because higher doses are nec-essary to make the microlaparoscopic procedure tolerable, the patient is unable to respond purposefully.

DEMEROL

Of the commonly used narcotics, Demerol probably has the least surgically useful analgesic properties for microlaparoscopic procedures. It has significant sedative hypnotic properties that further limit its utility. Other disadvantages include increased heart rate, decreased cardiac contractility, histamine release, and a long half-life.

SUFENTANIL

Sufentanil is similar to fentanyl, but more potent. It shares most of fentanyl's advantages and disadvantages. It has a smaller volume of distribution than fentanyl, and multiple doses or infusions of this drug make the analgesic: toxic ratio lower.

ALFENTANIL

As with sufentanil, alfentanil has similar properties to fentanyl. It has a shorter half-life and is a weaker agent than fentanyl. Its volume of distribution is small, so repeat dosing and/or infusions do not have as prolonged an effect. Major problems exist with alfentanil, especially with large doses; it can cause unconsciousness, marked nausea, and vomiting.

OPIOID AGONIST/ANTAGONIST AGENTS

The commonly used members of the opioid agonist/antagonist group include pentazocine, butorphanol, and nalbuphine. We prefer to avoid these agents, especially in conscious pain mapping procedures, because as a group they are more likely than Fentanyl to produce dysphoric responses. In addition, they can be quite sedating, causing significant nausea and vomiting, and are more difficult to reverse with naloxone than are the pure opioid agonists.

ANXIOLYTIC AGENTS

MIDAZOLAM

Midazolam is our anxiolytic agent of choice. It has replaced Valium for many endoscopic procedures because of its rapid onset of action, reversibility, and relatively short duration of action. Unlike Valium, it does not cause phlebitis along its injection course and does not cause pain when injected. In the past, an overdose of benzodiazepines was treated with supportive therapy until the drug wore off. Currently, the reversal agent of choice for midazolam is flumazenil, a specific benzodiazepine-receptor antagonist.

DIAZEPAM

Valium is the prototypical benzodiazepine to which others are compared. It exhibits potent anxiolytic properties and has hypnotic effects. Its use is limited by difficult parenteral administation, which causes phlebitis along its injection course and significant irritation upon injection. The drug is poorly soluble in intravenous fluids and can crystallize in intravenous lines. Its long half-life makes it a poor choice for office-based procedures. Comparable to the opioids, the benzodiazepines can be reversed. Flumazenil is the agent employed. Similar to Narcan and the opioids, flumazenil has a short half-life and repeat dosing is commonly required.

LORAZEPAM

We have found lorazepam to be of limited use. The drug is very potent, highly sedating, and has a relatively long duration of action. These are all undesirable properties for any drug employed in a conscious procedure.

NONSTEROIDAL ANTI-INFLAMMATORY DRUGS (NSAIDs)

KETOROLAC

Ketorolac is the only useful parenteral member of the NSAIDs. It has the advantage of analgesia without respiratory depression, sedation, or emesis. The drug has an opioid potency equivalence to about 5 to 10 mg of morphine, without any additive effects because it is non-narcotic. Unfortunately, the drug also exhibits side effects unique to its class of compounds: platelet inhibition, potential for bronchospasm, exacerbation of ulcerative disease, and renal toxicity. The latter is especially significant in patients who are volume contracted. The manufacturer recommends that a creatinine be checked and dosage lowered for levels of 1.5 mg/dL or greater. We have found this drug to be useful in relieving postoperative pain when administered toward the end of an operative microlaparoscopic procedure.

KETAMINE

Ketamine is a phencyclidine derivative and potent dissociative anesthetic with amnesic properties. It has no role in conscious pain mapping procedures and a limited role in office procedures such as tubal ligation. The problem encountered with this agent is delirium/dysphoria when used alone. The drug can produce unconsciousness when used in concert with midazolam. This is often followed by a milder delirium/dysphoria when the patient regains consciousness.

PROPOFOL

Propofol is a very short acting isopropylphenol derivative and a sedative hypnotic often used as an induction agent in place of pentothal. Hypnosis is produced rapidly and smoothly within 40 sec. It possesses many useful properties, acting as an antiemetic, antipruritic, and anxiolytic agent. The problem arises in that there is significant pain on injection and is highly sedating with a relatively small window of safety compared to midazolam. This limits its use for microlaparoscopic procedures under local anesthesia. In selected cases in which deep sedation is desirable, propofol is a good agent, especially for operative microlaparoscopic procedures.

LOCALLY ACTING AGENTS

Lidocaine with epinephrine is currently our agent of choice for local effects. When administered through a 27-gauge or smaller needle, it greatly minimizes patient discomfort during trocar insertion. The agent has a very rapid onset of action and provides some degree of postoperative analgesia as well. In addition to providing some degree of hemostasis, the epinephrine also prolongs the action of the lidocaine by producing vasospasm locally and permitting the drug to remain at its desired site. Sodium bicarbonate is mixed with lidocaine to decrease pain sensation during injection, owing to its buffering effect on pH. Marcaine is also commonly used. It has a slower onset of action than lidocaine, but a longer duration of action. For this reason, some surgeons use the two drugs together. Table 4.3 details our protocol for conscious sedation in microlaparoscopy.

TABLE 4-3. OUR PROTOCOL FOR CONSCIOUS SEDATION
IN MICROLAPAROSCOPY.[a]

- **Atropine:** 0.2 mg administered preoperatively to reduce the risk of a vasovagal reaction
- **Ondansetron hydrochloride (Zofran)[b]:** 4 mg to prevent nausea/vomiting
- **Midazolam hydrochloride (Versed)[b]:** 1–2 mg, *very rarely* 3 mg for a large patient
- **Fentanyl citrate[b]:** 250-μg administered *slowly* over 10 min and titrated in 50-μg increments to effect
- **Prophylactic antibiotic of choice**
- **1% lidocaine with epinephrine 1:100,000,[c]:** 10 mL buffered with sodium bicarbonate 10:1 dilution to decrease tissue irritation

---

[a]Almeida et al. (2)
[b]Administered intravenously.
[c]Administered intramuscularly or paracerucally.

COMMENTS

Our protocol for conscious sedation in microlaparoscopy was developed out of frustration with existing protocols in the literature. For example, one protocol used 5 mg midazolam which produces too much sedation, especially for conscious pain mapping and maximum doses of fentanyl at 100-μg, which does not provide adequate pain relief. To date, when using our protocol, we have not had a single case in which the patient required intubation, bagging by mask, or use of reversal agents; and none had an oxygen saturation <94%. No woman experienced hypotension, tachycardia, nausea, vomiting, or dyspnea. In selected patients, this protocol has allowed us to perform diagnostic microlaparoscopy, including conscious pain mapping (2,4,5); operative microlaparoscopy, including primary lysis of adhesions (2,4,6); fulguration of endometriosis (2,4,6); laparoscopic uterosacral nerve ablation (4,6); drainage of ovarian cysts (4); appendectomy (7); and ovarian drilling (8).

REFERENCES

1. Peterson HB, DeStefano F, Rubin GL, et al. Deaths attributable to tubal sterilization in the United States, 1977 to 1981. Am J Obstet Gynecol 146:131–136, 1983.

2. Almeida OD Jr, Val-Gallas JM, Browning JL. A protocol for conscious sedation in microlaparoscopy. J Am Assoc Gynecol Laparosc 4:591–594, 1997.

3. American Society of Anesthesiologists. Practice guidelines for sedation and analgesia by non-anesthesiologists. Anesth 84:459–471, 1996.

4. Almeida OD Jr, Val-Gallas JM. Conscious pain mapping. J Am Assoc Gynecol Laparosc 4:587–590, 1997.

5. Almeida OD Jr, Val-Gallas JM, Rizk B. A novel classification for conscious pain mapping. Egy. J Fertil Steril 1:53–58, 1997.

6. Almeida OD Jr, Val-Gallas JM. Office microlaparoscopy under local anesthesia in the diagnosis and treatment of chronic pelvic pain. J Am Assoc Gynecol Laparosc 5:407–410, 1998.

7. Almeida OD Jr, Val-Gallas JM, Rizk B. Appendectomy under local anesthesia following conscious pain mapping with microlaparoscopy. Hum Reprod 13:588–590, 1998.

8. Almeida OD Jr, Rizk B. Microlaparoscopic ovarian drilling under local anesthesia. Middle East Fertil Soc J 3:189–191, 1998.

PATIENT SELECTION AND PREOPERATIVE COUNSELING

JOHN M. VAL-GALLAS, M.D., F.A.C.O.G., F.A.C.S.

PATIENT SELECTION

Appropriate patient selection is critical to the performance of safe office-based surgery. Only a segment of patients who are otherwise suitable outpatient surgical candidates can be considered for in-office laparoscopy. The aim of careful patient selection is to reduce patient risk and at the same time identify which women are good candidates for these minimally invasive office procedures.

The preoperative evaluation is the single most important factor involved in the prevention of complications. This includes a complete history, physical examination, and appropriate laboratory testing. More potential problems and previously undiagnosed disorders are identified by the history and physical examination than by laboratory testing. We strictly limit our office microlaparoscopic procedures to patients whose physical status places them at an American Society of Anesthesiologists (ASA) level 1 or 2. This effectively eliminates patients with problems such as poorly controlled cardiac or respiratory disease, neuropathic or swallowing disorders and patients with chronic debilitating hepatic or renal disease.

The patient's past surgical history is also a consideration, especially if there is mention of a prior procedure with intestinal spill or infection. Often these patients are best served by having their procedure done in a traditional operating room. The type of previous abdominal incision may expose a patient to some degree of increased risk of complications associated with bowel injury. The risk of anterior abdominal wall adhesions to bowel or omentum is higher with vertical incisions than with Pfannenstiel incisions. History of a prior cesarean section produces less concern, because the

Microlaparoscopy, Edited by Oscar D. Almeida, Jr.
ISBN 0-471-34574-1   Copyright © 2000 by Wiley-Liss, Inc.

slowly involuting uterus protects the anterior abdominal wall from adhesion formation to some degree by displacing the bowel and omentum. Infections and multiple prior surgeries, however, still increase the risk of uterine adherence, regardless of incision type.

Patient weight can be a relative contraindication to office laparoscopy. There is no absolute upper weight limit, depending on surgeon experience; however, body habitus is important. Patients with a prior term pregnancy usually have a more flaccid abdominal wall and are better surgical candidates than women who have not given birth at term. Also, patients with a lean panniculus and/or thin area under the abdominal curvature make peritoneal entry relatively simple. A thick abdominal wall can make insufflation difficult to perform. Surgeons are currently limited to one trocar length with the available instrumentation. There is an increased likelihood of bending a delicate microlaparoscope, particularly when viewing at acute angles in the morbidly obese patient.

The patient's airway is another significant anatomic consideration. We avoid doing office-based microlaparoscopy on patients with other than a class I or II airway. Fortunately, seizures and anaphylaxis are relatively rare events. Adverse drug reactions can occur and have the potential to compromise a patient's airway. Prior anesthetic experiences of the patient, allergies and any difficulties with anesthesia encountered by close relatives of the patient should be addressed. A patient's own home medications also become important, because many prescription drugs may have antagonistic or synergistic effects in combination with the agents employed in conscious sedation protocols.

The patient's differential diagnosis must be weighed when deciding whether a procedure can be safely performed in the office. Patients with an ileus or large complex pelvic mass could potentially have laparoscopic surgery but are at a relatively greater risk of requiring a laparotomy under general anesthesia. A traditional operating room would be a more suitable theater for such individuals. Office microlaparoscopic procedures are most appropriate for diagnoses and treatment of such entities as chronic pelvic pain, undesired fertility, simple cysts, infertility evaluations, and other nonemergent situations.

Psychiatric history and patient motivation are of paramount importance when contemplating an office microlaparoscopy. Any active psychiatric illness is a relative contraindication to office-based surgery. These patients are frequently on similar agents to those used in conscious sedation. Drug tolerance to high doses of benzodiazepines or opiates is commonly seen. At the drug levels required for effect in these patients, the therapeutic:toxic ratio is dangerously low. Therefore, former or recovering addicts are not considered candidates for conscious procedures.

Other special situations include patients at the extremes of age, the mentally challenged, the hearing impaired, and those with a primary language other than English (or the surgeon's native tongue). Increased anxiety when encountering new situations is difficult to predict. Accordingly, we have found the "belly test" (by which the abdominal skin is grasped and lifted at the preoperative visit to determine whether the patient is a good candidate for a conscious procedure) to be of limited usefulness when using our office protocol (1). Most patients who experience discomfort with the belly test preoperatively, still tolerate the procedures well. It has been our experience that the majority of our patients have been interested in conscious procedures, well motivated, and even enthusiastic about participating in their own care.

PREOPERATIVE COUNSELING

Preoperative counseling of the patient is more extensive and detail-oriented for a conscious procedure than for one performed under general anesthesia. During counseling, one must keep in mind that the patient will experience all phases of the procedure. This includes the preparation, positioning, draping, surgery, and recovery. During this time, she will also be fully cognizant and interactive with the surgical team. The usual surgical preoperative counseling regarding risks, benefits, alternatives, and possible complications must be supplemented for office-based laparoscopic procedures. First, the patient should be given the opportunity to choose her desired method of anesthesia and site of procedure. For example, office procedures done under conscious sedation vs. hospital or ambulatory surgery center with conscious sedation or general anesthesia. Patients should be informed of the limitations involving conscious procedures, office-based procedures, and laparoscopic procedures in general. For example, general anesthesia is usually not available in the office setting and an unplanned emergency laparotomy may need to be done under local anesthesia. Should an elective operative microlaparoscopic procedure become too uncomfortable for the patient, it will not be completed in the office. When a surgical procedure does not appear to be technically feasible in the office, only the diagnostic portion of the procedure will be performed.

Patients like to maintain control of their situation as much as possible. Most have never seen the inside of an operating room. Ideally, members of the surgical team should be introduced to the patient, their roles described, and the type of contact they will have discussed during the preoperative counseling session. Abdominal and vaginal preparations, positioning, draping, Foley catheter insertion, and monitoring devices should all be explained to the patient before the procedure.

For a conscious procedure, the surgeon must review the surgical portion of the case with the patient in a step-by-step fashion. After all, it is this portion of the procedure that will cause the most discomfort to the patient and likely provoke the majority of questions. Topics to discuss include the placement of a uterine manipulator, use of local and intravenous medications in addition to what effects the medicines will have, grasping of the abdominal wall, Veress needle and trocar insertion, CO_2 insufflation, Trendelenburg position, and probing of structures. The patient needs to know that she should expect some discomfort associated with the procedure, but she will be informed of what is happening during the surgery and when to expect different sensations.

The postoperative recovery period merits advance discussion for all microlaparoscopic procedures. This should include monitoring, recovery time, and tasks that a patient must perform before discharge. Discharge teaching must address home limitations, driving, wound care, general warnings, medications, and follow-up appointment. The patient should be given a general understanding of problems that may occur, when to call emergently, and when to call non-emergently. An adult should be ready to be responsible for the patient's care when she is discharged.

REFERENCES

1. Almeida OD Jr, Val-Gallas JM. A protocol for conscious sedation in microlaparoscopy. J Am Assoc Gynecol Laparosc 4:591–594, 1997.

DIAGNOSTIC MICROLAPAROSCOPY

OSCAR D. ALMEIDA, JR., M.D., F.A.C.O.G., F.A.C.S.

Patients with indeterminate findings after a thorough physical examination and laboratory workup, including a transvaginal ultrasound, may be candidates for a diagnostic microlaparoscopy. In selected patients, microlaparoscopy under local anesthesia with conscious sedation is an acceptable alternative to traditional laparoscopy under general anesthesia. Although general anesthesia is appropriate for lengthy or complex procedures, most diagnostic microlaparoscopic cases can be easily and safely performed under local anesthesia with conscious sedation (1). Microlaparoscopy should be considered when traditional laparoscopy may be contraindicated, particularly in patients with previous multiple abdominal surgeries.

Every gynecologist who performs laparoscopic surgery should add the technique of diagnostic microlaparoscopy under local anesthesia to his or her armamentarium. This minimally invasive surgical procedure requires formal training and new learning, even for the expert laparoscopist. Two important factors should be considered. First, most gynecologists are unfamiliar with the new delicate microinstrumentation and its use. Second, it is a totally different experience performing laparoscopy on an awake patient.

Microlaparoscopy under local anesthesia provides a rapid, minimally invasive glance at pelvic and abdominal structures. This information is now more accessible to the physician and patient, because microlaparoscopy can be done in the physician's office or ambulatory surgery center. Whereas diagnostic methods such as ultrasound may not identify the etiology of pain due to endometriosis or adhesions, a definitive diagnosis is possible in many cases using this technique.

Diagnostic possibilities consist of both nonemergent and emergent conditions. These are summarized in Table 6.1. Acute pelvic pain of uncertain etiology can be evaluated with microlaparoscopy under local anesthesia to

Microlaparoscopy, Edited by Oscar D. Almeida Jr.
ISBN 0-471-34574-1   Copyright © 2000 by Wiley-Liss, Inc.

TABLE 6.1. CONDITIONS EVALUATED USING DIAGNOSTIC
MICROLAPAROSCOPY UNDER LOCAL ANESTHESIA

- Evaluating pelvic pain (conscious pain mapping)
- Diagnosing endometriosis
- Diagnosing pelvic adhesions
- Evaluating infertility (chromotubation)
- Monitoring ectopic pregnancy being treated with methotrexate
- Evaluating right lower quadrant pain (acute appendicitis; other chronic abnormalities of the appendix)
- Diagnosing hemorrhagic ovarian cysts
- Diagnosing pelvic inflammatory disease

differentiate between cases such as pelvic inflammatory disease, early appendicitis, adnexal torsion, or a ruptured, ovarian cyst. Another avenue readily available with this technique includes second-look microlaparoscopy, an important adjunct to continued surveillance in certain conditions such as pelvic adhesions. Patients who elect medical therapy with methotrexate for an ectopic pregnancy will occassionally experience pain as a result of necrosis of the villi. In this situation, the pain is difficult to differentiate from rupture of the tubal pregnancy. Microlaparoscopy under local anesthesia can be employed for diagnosis in this situation and possibly prevent the need for a procedure under general anesthesia.

The single most important aspect of diagnostic microlaparoscopy under local anesthesia for the clinician to keep in mind is that the patient is awake throughout the entire procedure. Unlike traditional laparoscopy in which the patient is asleep under general anesthesia, the clinician can communicate directly with the patient and obtain feedback from her during surgery. Patient selection, comfort, and good communication are vital for success. Impending bodily contact should be conveyed to the patient each time.

POSITIONING THE PATIENT

With traditional laparoscopy, the patient is positioned for surgery following induction of general anesthesia. In contradistinction during microlaparoscopy under local anesthesia, at the beginning of the case the patient is placed in the dorso-lithotomy position using behind-the-knee stirrups (Fig. 6.1). Attention should be paid to her comfort before starting any other aspect of the procedure. Repositioning the patient may provoke anxiety which can be reduced by making sure she is down far enough on the table. The Trendelenburg position is used as necessary to facilitate visualization of the pelvis.

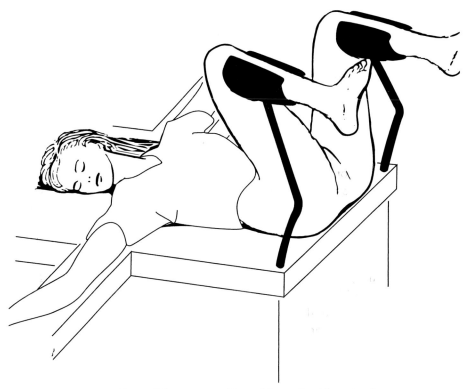

FIGURE 6.1. Dorso-lithotomy position of the patient for microlaparoscopy.

PREPARING AND MONITORING THE PATIENT

The patient is asked to use a Fleet enema the night before surgery as a bowel evacuant to allow better visualization of the pelvic and abdominal cavities during microlaparoscopy. All patients should be fasting a minimum of 7 h. After starting an intravenous line with Ringer's lactate solution, oxygen via nasal cannula is administered. Patient monitoring includes the use of a continuous ECG, heart rate, and respiratory monitors; pulseoximeter, and automated blood pressure cuff. Monitors that simultaneously provide these functions are ideal. Data obtained should be charted appropriately, at least every 5 min.

Once the patient is properly positioned on the operating table, the skin is sterily prepared and draped. Although a few clinicians do not routinely use a Foley catheter for pelvic surgery, we highly recommend its use during microlaparoscopy to reduce the risk of bladder injury. Bladder injury during laparoscopy is more common in patients with previous pelvic surgery than in those without such surgery. Viscous lidocaine may be applied when inserting the Foley catheter to decrease the patient's discomfort.

The optimum drug combination is critical for the procedure, because its success lies in the balance of patient comfort. We have employed many intravenous drug combinations recommended by physicians who perform laparoscopic tubal ligations under local anesthesia and found the results disappointing when used for diagnostic and operative microlaparoscopy. The drugs produced either too much sedation, too little pain relief, or both. The goal is to make the patient comfortable while remaining lucid.

The administration of drugs should be based on the patient's weight, and doses titrated in a methodical manner to ensure patient safety and satisfactory levels of sedation and analgesia. Preoperatively, the patient is given 0.2 mg atropine to decrease the risk of a vasovagal reaction, 4 mg Zofran for prevention of nausea, and 1 to 2 mg Versed (midazolam) for sedation. Before starting the procedure, the patient receives a total of 250 µg of fentanyl *slowly*, which is then titrated to effect. We have had patients who required up to 500 µg of fentanyl in order to comfortably perform the diagnostic microlaparoscopy. *Continuous careful monitoring of the patient, especially the respiratory rate, cannot be overemphasized* (2). It is at this point that the physician or nurse monitoring the patient may occasionally need to remind the patient to take in a deep breath.

We use 10 mL of 1% lidocaine with epinephrine 1:100,000 as the local anesthetic. It is buffered with sodium bicarbonate in a 10:1 dilution to decrease tissue irritation when administered for both the paracervical block before placement of a uterine manipulator of choice and the umbilical block at the site of a 2-mm cannula placement. The cervical block is administered in a clockwise manner to include the entire cervix. Following an initial vertical skin block that penetrates the abdominal wall, four additional blocks are placed at 45° angles to the vertical tract in a north, south, east, and west fashion (Fig. 6.2). All skin blocks are administered without removal of the needle until the block is completed. Especially in very thin patients, it is prudent to elevate the abdominal wall in order to prevent injury to the underlying structures.

INSERTING THE VERESS NEEDLE WITH THE TROCAR AND CREATING A PNEUMOPERITONEUM

Using the microlaparoscope allows for a much safer access into the abdominal cavity than using a large diameter trocar. A 2-mm umbilical incision is made using a #11 scalpel blade. Figure 6.3 outlines trocar placement sites. The Veress needle and 2-mm trocar sheath are simultaneously introduced transumbilically into the abdominal cavity for visual access after elevating the abdominal skin (Fig. 6.4).

Patency of the Veress needle is checked using the *saline drop test*. Once patency is established, a pneumoperitoneum is created. We prefer using carbon dioxide as the pneumoperitoneum medium in the event that operative microlaparoscopy is necessary. Table 6.2 details the advantages and disadvantages of carbon dioxide. Nitrous oxide can be used, but it reportedly carries a small risk of combustion (3). Other surgeons have reported a

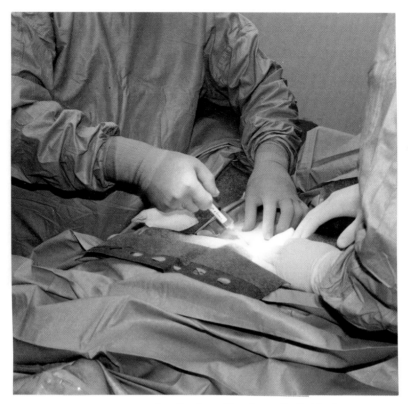

FIGURE 6.2. Application of local anesthetic block.

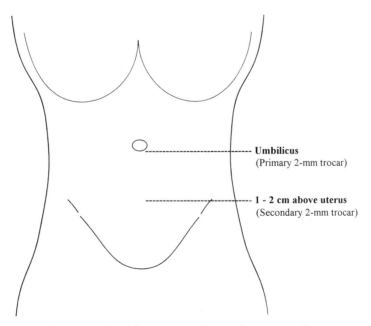

FIGURE 6.3. Sites of primary and secondary trocar placement.

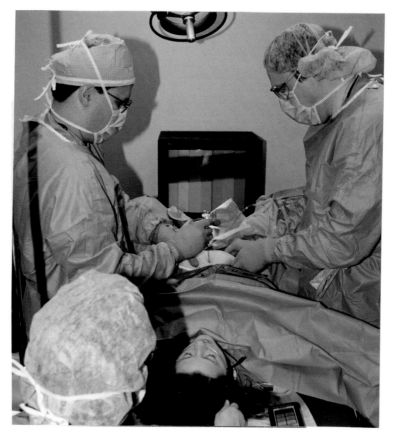

FIGURE 6.4. Elevation of the abdomen before trocar and Veress needle insertion.

TABLE 6.2. USE OF CARBON DIOXIDE IN MICROLAPAROSCOPY

Advantages

- Preferred gas for the creation of pneumoperitoneum
- Inexpensive
- Rapidly eliminated
- Known to suppress combustion
- Readily absorbed

Disadvantages

- Hypercarbia
- Respiratory acidosis
- Tachycardia
- Cardiac arrhythmias
- Peritoneal irritation
- Decreased stroke volume

TABLE 6.3. USE OF NITROUS OXIDE IN MICROLAPAROSCOPY

Advantages

- Inexpensive
- Rapidly absorbed
- Rapidly eliminated
- Has anesthetic effects
- Lacks the hemodynamic side effects of carbon dioxide
- May be beneficial for prolonged cases

Disadvantages

- Does not suppress combustion

preference for nitrous oxide or room air and state that there are no adverse accounts when cauterizing for hemostasis specifically related to the presence of nitrous oxide (4). Table 6.3 summarizes the pros and cons of nitrous oxide.

We have noted that the volume of gas tolerated by the awake patient varies. 1.5 L of CO_2 is usually well tolerated and allows for excellent visualization of the pelvic cavity, thus serving as an excellent starting point for these cases. The volume of CO_2 is inversely proportional to the length of time that the patient will tolerate a microlaparoscopic procedure under local anesthesia due to peritoneal irritation. For example, using a small volume of CO_2 such as 1.5 L will allow for a longer procedure. We have observed that patients tolerate procedures lasting up to 2.5 h. comfortably with these small volumes. On the other hand, after 30 min many patients with 2.5 L experience peritoneal irritation. On occasion, the morbidly obese patient may require up to 3 L CO_2. The patient should be told before surgery that she may experience a sensation of extreme abdominal fullness and pressure under her diaphragm resulting from the pneumoperitoneum. Knowing this ahead of time will help decrease her level of anxiety. Intra-abdominal pressures of CO_2 8 mm Hg will usually result in patient discomfort during awake procedures.

PERFORMING DIAGNOSTIC MICROLAPAROSCOPY

Once the pneumoperitoneum is created, the 2-mm microlaparoscope is inserted. After visually identifying an appropriate suprapubic landmark and infiltrating it with local anesthesia in the same fashion as the umbilical block was performed, a 2-mm trocar is inserted under direct visualization and a manipulating probe inserted. We use a probe marked in centimeters to assist in measuring the fallopian tube length in cases in which tubal anastomosis is being considered and in estimating the size of lesion (See Fig. 3.4, **A**).

Once all instruments are in place and the patient is in the Trendelenburg position, diagnostic microlaparoscopy through a systematic visual examination of the pelvic and abdominal cavities is performed. It is important to remember that operating time should be kept to a minimum because the patient is awake. Note that 1% lidocaine without epinephrine can be applied directly to any area of discomfort, because it is readily absorbed through peritoneal surfaces. When indicated, chromotubation is conducted at this time.

FINISHING THE PROCEDURE

Postoperative chest and shoulder pain may result from the residual CO_2 pneumoperitoneum. Once the procedure is completed, an effort to eliminate as much of the gas medium is made *while the patient is still in the Trendelenburg position* before removing the trocars. Post-operative instructions should include mention of possible shoulder pain due to any remaining gas. The incision sites are approximated with Steri-strips to optimize the aesthetic appearence once they are healed. No sutures are required! When the patient is fully alert, which is generally immediately following the procedure, the patient is given liquids orally.

The patient is recovered and monitored on the operating table. At this time, the video and operative findings can be reviewed and discussed in detail with the patient and her partner. Under most circumstances, the patient should be able to walk out of the office fully recovered within 1h after completion of the procedure. It is recommended that reversal agents not be used unless there are specific circumstances, such as respiratory depression.

Our general sense of the applicability of this approach is that many procedures done as traditional laparoscopy under general anesthesia could be done in a less invasive manner. As advances continue to be made with both microlaparoscopic techniques and instrumentation, this protocol will assist clinicians in diagnostic and operative microlaparoscopy.

REFERENCES

1. Almeida OD Jr, Val-Gallas JM. Office microlaparoscopy under local anesthesia in the diagnosis and treatment of chronic pelvic pain. J Am Assoc Gynecol Laparosc. 5:407–410, 1998.
2. Almeida OD Jr, Val-Gallas JM and Browning JL. A protocol for conscious sedation in micro-laparoscopy. J Am Assoc Gynecol Laparosc 4:591–594, 1997.
3. Neuman GG, Sidebotham G, Negoianu E, et al. Laparoscopy explosion hazards with nitrous oxide. Anesth.78:875–879, 1993.
4. Penfield AJ. Laparoscopy for diagnosis or sterilization. In Penfield AJ, ed. Outpatient gynecologic surgery. Baltimore:Williams & Wilkins, 1997:136–137.

CONSCIOUS PAIN MAPPING

OSCAR D. ALMEIDA, JR., M.D., F.A.C.O.G., F.A.C.S.

Traditional laparoscopy for the evaluation of chronic pelvic pain has a major flaw. Until recently, this diagnostic gold standard has had clinicians addressing lesions visible through the laparoscope to investigate the etiology of their patient's pain. The primary limitation of the procedure has always been the use of general anesthesia, which does not allow for intraoperative patient feedback. Unfortunately, not all visible lesions such as endometriosis and adhesions, account for all of the patient's symptoms.(1–3). In addition, deep lesions may exist that are not readily visible through the laparoscope and can be missed if the procedure is performed under general anesthesia (1).

Conscious pain mapping has added an innovative diagnostic dimension previously absent in gynecology.(1,4). Because she is awake for the entire microlaparoscopic procedure, the patient can provide crucial information as an active member of the surgical team by helping the surgeon locate the source of her pain. The ability to identify and reproduce pain in the area(s) of the pelvic and abdominal cavities that have caused the patient her discomfort is the hallmark of conscious pain mapping.

Chronic pelvic pain is defined as pain that has lasted 6 months or longer and is severe enough to affect a woman's daily functioning and personal relationships. These symptoms are usually unresolved with conservative medical therapy, such as oral contraceptives, NSAIDs, and antibiotics when appropriate. Changes in appetite, weight loss, and sleep disturbances are common. Nongynecologic causes of chronic pelvic pain must be ruled out (Table 7.1). When localized pelvic pain is present for at least 6 months, the diagnostic yield at laparoscopy is increased. Additional data obtained by conscious pain mapping assist in providing a more thorough evaluation than traditional laparoscopy under general anesthesia.

Microlaparoscopy, Edited by Oscar D. Almeida, Jr.
ISBN 0-471-34574-1   Copyright © 2000 by Wiley-Liss, Inc.

TABLE 7.1. NONGYNECOLOGIC ORIGINS OF CHRONIC PELVIC PAIN

Urinary tract
Gastrointestinal tract
Musculoskeletal
Neurologic
Psychologic

Chronic pelvic pain accounts for approximately 10 to 15% of a woman's visits to the gynecologist, up to 50% of diagnostic laparoscopies, and many hysterectomies each year. (5). Interestingly, 10 to 60% of patients have no pathologic findings using the traditional laparoscopic approach under general anesthesia. Physical examination sometimes provides confusing and minimal useful data for the evaluation of chronic pelvic pain. In a large study of 1194 patients with chronic pelvic pain, normal pelvic examinations were found in 749 patients (6). Not surprisingly, in 479 of patients with chronic pelvic pain and a normal examination, 63% had abnormal findings during diagnostic laparoscopy. However, 17.5% of the study patients with an abnormal pelvic examination had a normal diagnostic laparoscopy. It is for this latter subgroup of patients that conscious pain mapping may provide more clinical information than with traditional laparoscopy.

Most staging of endometriosis is related to infertility rather than pelvic pain. It is difficult to evaluate the severity of pelvic pain using the revised American Fertility Society (AFS) classification of endometriosis. (7,8). The primary limitation with this classification is that there is no consistent relationship between the severity of endometriosis and pelvic pain. For example, a patient with the AFS stage IV endometriosis may have mild tenderness and one with stage I minimal disease can have severe, excruciating symptoms. A recent AFS (now the American Society for Reproductive Medicine) classification of endometriosis in the presence of pelvic pain describes the patient's symptoms of pelvic pain. (9). The intraoperative component of this evaluation, however, is performed while the patient is asleep under general anesthesia. Conscious pain mapping cannot be done under general anesthesia because the patient must be awake for the procedure.

CONSCIOUS PAIN MAPPING (CPM)

The technique of diagnostic microlaparoscopy under local anesthesia with conscious sedation was outlined in Chapter 6 (1,10); visual data obtained through the microlaparoscope are combined with pain sensations reported by the patient as the pelvic and abdominal cavities are systematically probed. It is important to position the cannula 1 to 2 cm cephalic to the uterine fundus to avoid placing excess pressure by the probe when elevating the uterus to evaluate the cul-de-sac. By inserting the needle into the pelvis for the local anesthetic block (Fig. 7.1), the surgeon can identify the

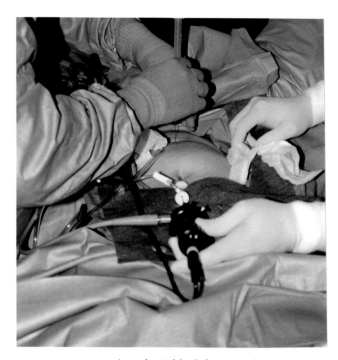

FIGURE 7.1. Anesthetic block for secondary trocar.

appropriate location for trocar placement (Fig. 7.2). A 2-mm blunt probe introduced through a cannula in the suprapubic region is used for this function (Fig. 7.3). Gentle probing is maintained long enough to elicit a response. Figure 7.4 illustrates the *minimum* sequence employed for pain mapping. If several lesions are seen on a single organ (endometriosis, adhesions, scarring), each lesion is probed systematically. The uterus is not elevated in the early part of the procedure, to avoid eliciting unnecessary painful stimuli.

The findings are then mapped on a diagram of the pelvic cavity. Painful areas are probed a second time to authenticate their roles as pain foci. These results are graded on a scale of 0 to 4, and a mean score is assigned (11), which is classified as absent, minimal, mild, moderate, or severe. (Fig. 7.5) Unlike using a grading system of 1 to 100 or even 1 to 10, we believe that this system is more physician/patient friendly and makes it easier to obtain intraoperative feedback from the patient who is under conscious sedation. Before surgery, it is imperative to educate and familiarize the patient with the procedure, what you are trying to accomplish, and the grading system.

A score of 0 means that the area probed produced no pain. The patient is asked to define severe pain, graded with a score of 4, as that pain which if always present would be crippling. Moderate, mild, and minimal pain—graded as 3, 2, and 1, respectively—are described on a declining scale. Because some pelvic structures such as an ovary or appendix may be surgically absent, a mean score is obtained only for the evaluated areas and an overall pain classification assigned.

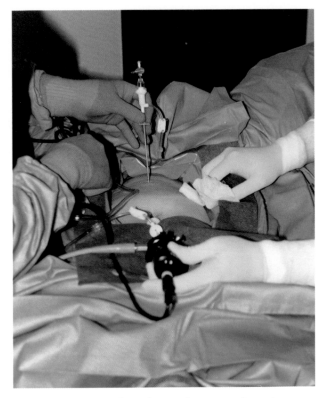

FIGURE 7.2. Site of secondary trocar insertion.

Our preliminary study using the technique of conscious pain mapping revealed that significant adhesions are often associated with pelvic pain as are at times subtle lesions, which may be overlooked if the procedure is done under general anesthesia without patient feedback (1). Reproduction of pelvic pain by probing the endometriosis lesions was inconsistent, regardless of lesion size or location, and some were entirely nontender. A total of 80.6% of the women with severe pelvic adhesions had tenderness to manipulation of adhesions during pain mapping. The most significant finding of that study was the role of the appendix in chronic pelvic pain. We noted a yield of 69.2% abnormal pathologic findings of the appendix when the appendix was severely tender or appeared anatomically distorted. Table 7.2 summarizes the abnormal appendix findings.

The preliminary findings were consistent with a subsequent study that revealed that 70% of women who underwent an appendectomy after evaluation of the appendix with conscious pain mapping had abnormal pathologic findings compared to 24% of patients who had an incidental appendectomy (12). These results suggest that conscious pain mapping of the appendix in women with chronic pelvic pain assists the clinician in identifying which patients should undergo an appendectomy so that an incidental appendectomy need not be performed on all patients with chronic pelvic pain.

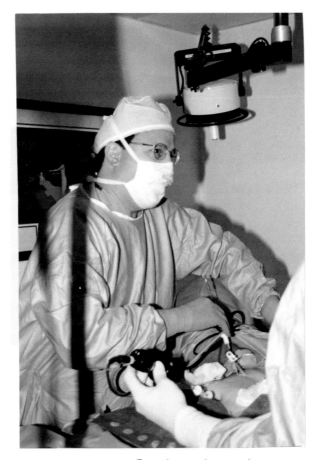

FIGURE 7.3. Conscious pain mapping.

More recently, two intriguing case reports combining superior hypogastric plexus block with pain mapping were presented. (13). This technique is used to more properly select which women may benefit from a presacral neurectomy. After conscious pain mapping, local anesthesia is injected into the presacral retroperitoneal space. After 3 to 4 min, pain mapping is repeated. If the hypogastric block eliminates the pain, the patient with advanced endometriosis may experience amelioration of the central component of menstrual-associated pelvic pain after a presacral neurectomy.

TABLE 7.2. ABNORMAL APPENDIX FINDINGS

Findings	Number of Patients
Endometriosis	2
Focal acute appendicitis	1
Fecalith	2
Lymphoid hyperplasia	3
Fibrous obliteration of lumen	1
Severe periappendiceal adhesions	7

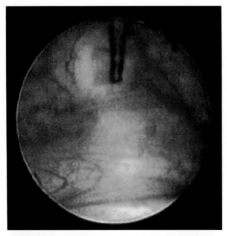

A, Probing the bladder.

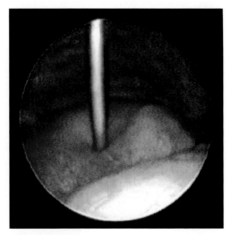

B, Probing the uterus.

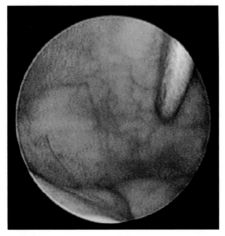

C, Probing the posterior cul-de-sac.

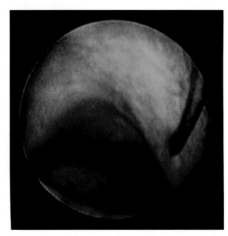

D, Probing the right uterosacral ligament.

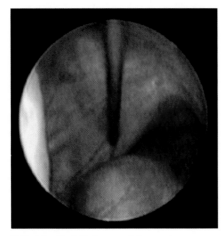

E, Probing the left uterosacral ligament.

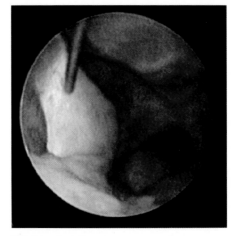

F, Probing the left ovary.

FIGURE 7.4. Minimum probing sequence for conscious pain mapping.

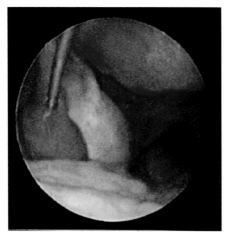

G, Probing the left fallopian tube.

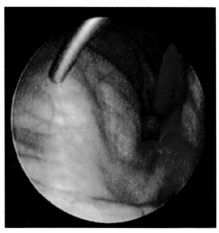

H, Probing the left pelvic sidewall.

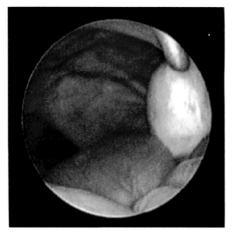

I, Probing the right ovary.

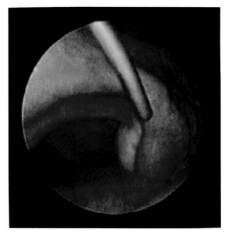

J, Probing the right fallopian tube.

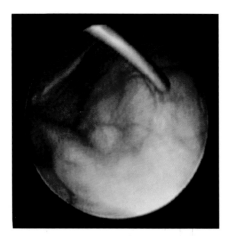

K, Probing the right pelvic sidewall.

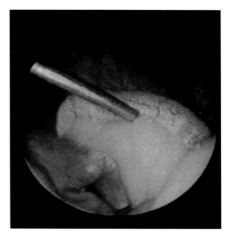

I, Probing the appendix.

CLASSIFICATION OF CONSCIOUS PAIN MAPPING

Patient's Name _____ Age ____ Date of Birth _____ Date _____

Site	Score	Comments
Bladder		
Uterus		
Posterior cul-de-sac		
Right uterosacral ligament		
Left uterosacral ligament		
Left ovary		
Left fallopian tube		
Left pelvic sidewall		
Right ovary		
Right fallopian tube		
Right pelvic sidewall		
Appendix		
TOTAL		
MEAN SCORE		

Pain Classification	Score
Absent	0
Minimal	1
Mild	2
Moderate	3
Severe	4

Comments _____

FIGURE 7.5. An intraoperative instrument to document the degree of chronic pelvic pain during conscious pain mapping

We have observed that the degree of pain relief in our patients has not been related as much to the amount of disease treated as to the specific site at which pain could be reproduced. For example, all of the women who underwent an appendectomy in our preliminary study experienced amelioration of their right lower quadrant pelvic pain. There were two appendices that appeared anatomically distorted secondary to fecaliths and should have been identified with traditional laparoscopy under general anesthesia. The remaining cases, however, would have been missed by traditional laparoscopy under general anesthesia, because those appendices appeared grossly normal.

A study in which only symptomatic lesions were treated might shed further light on the surgical management of patients with chronic pelvic pain. If pain relief after treatment of these specific lesions is significant, then the extent of surgery could be further limited, thus decreasing patient surgical risk and morbidity. It is unknown, however, if a nontender lesion today will become tender 6 months from now. In addition, this limited surgical approach would be applicable only to women with undesired fertility.

In summary, the goal of conscious pain mapping is to identify and reproduce pain in the area(s) of the patient's discomfort. Our conscious pain mapping classification provides a simple physician/patient friendly system of classification for pain mapping. As the uses for pain mapping continue to surge, we anticipate that more clinicians will use this technique for evaluation of selected women with chronic pelvic pain.

REFERENCES

1. Almeida OD Jr, Val-Gallas JM. Conscious pain mapping. J Am Assoc Gynecol Laparosc 4:587–590, 1997.

2. Demco L. Mapping the source and character of pain due to endometriosis by patient-assisted laparoscopy. J Am Assoc Gynecol Laparosc 5: 241–245, 1998.

3. Rapkin AJ. Adhesions and pelvic pain: a retrospective study. Obstet Gynecol 68:13–15, 1986.

4. Palter S, Olive D. Office microlaparoscopy under local anesthesia for chronic pelvic pain. J Am Assoc Gynecol Laparosc 3: 359–364, 1996.

5. Reiter R. A profile of women with chronic pelvic pain. Clin Obstet Gynecol 33: 130–136, 1990.

6. Cunanan RG, Courey NG, Lippes J. Laparoscopic findings in patients with pelvic pain. Am J Obstet Gynecol 146: 589–591, 1983.

7. Fukaya T, Hoshiai H, Yajima A. Is pelvic endometriosis always associated with chronic pain? A retrospective study of 618 cases diagnosed by laparoscopy. Am J Obstet Gynecol 169: 719–722, 1993.

8. American Fertility Society. Revised American Fertility Society classification of endometriosis: 1985. Fertil Steril 43:351–352, 1985.

9. American Fertility Society. Management of endometriosis in the presence of pelvic pain. Fertil Steril 60:952–955, 1993.

10. Almeida OD Jr, Val-Gallas JM, Browning JL. A protocol for conscious sedation in microlaparoscopy. J Am Assoc Gynecol Laparosc 4:591–594, 1997.

11. Almeida OD Jr, Val-Gallas JM, Rizk B. A novel classification for conscious pain mapping. Egy J Fertil Steril 1:53–58, 1997.

12. Almeida OD Jr, Val-Gallas JM. Conscious pain mapping of the appendix with microlaparoscopy for the evaluation of women with chronic pelvic pain. Mid East Fert Soc J, in press.

13. Steege JF. Superior hypogastric block during microlaparoscopic pain mapping. J Am Assoc Gynecol Laparosc 5:265–267, 1998.

OPERATIVE MICROLAPAROSCOPY

OSCAR D. ALMEIDA, JR., M.D., F.A.C.O.G., F.A.C.S.

Many surgical advances have been achieved since 1933 when Fervers first reported performing operative laparoscopy (1). He lysed adhesions and performed several intra-abdominal biopsies. During the 1990s, most operative gynecologic procedures previously done only via laparotomy have been performed with laparoscopy. More recently, the concept of minimally invasive surgery has continued to evolve.

Operative microlaparoscopy under local anesthesia is in its pioneer stage. Several laparoscopic procedures previously reported under general anesthesia can be safely and effectively performed under local anesthesia with conscious sedation in selected patients. These include electrosurgery for the fulguration of endometriosis (2,3), primary lysis of adhesions (2,3), laparoscopic uterosacral nerve ablation (LUNA) (2,3), appendectomy (4), and ovarian drilling.(5).

Many laparoscopic surgeries requiring general anesthesia are accomplished in a more minimally invasive fashion whenever microinstrumentation is incorporated into the procedure. An example is laparoscopic-assisted vaginal hysterectomies (LAVHs). Using a 2-mm microlaparoscope placed transumbilically, two additional 2-mm trocars are placed lateral to the rectus muscles. After placing the microlaparoscope in either lateral cannula, the 2-mm trocar in the umbilicus is replaced with an expandable 12-mm STEP trocar (InnerDyne Inc., Sunnyvale, CA), which is used to accommodate staple guns or tripolar scissors for the pedicles (Fig. 8.1). Regardless of the case, I always use the 2-mm microlaparoscope for the entire surgical procedure and do not change to a larger laparoscope.

The advantages of this combined approach are threefold. First, patients appear to have minimal postoperative pain and discomfort in sites where a smaller cannula is used, due to less tissue damage. Second, the aesthetic

Microlaparoscopy, Edited by Oscar D. Almeida Jr.
ISBN 0-471-34574-1   Copyright © 2000 by Wiley-Liss, Inc.

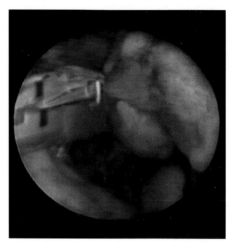

FIGURE 8.1. Microlaparoscopic LAVH
using a linear stapling device.

results are superior with the 2-mm trocars compared to the 10- or 12-mm
trocars at any location other than the umbilicus or lower pelvis. Unfortunately, we have all seen these avoidable deforming scars. Finally, the
incision site(s) of 2-mm trocars do not require suturing.

The only technical limitation that I have encountered with operative
microlaparoscopy is that in certain procedures, (e.g., during appendectomies, LAVHs and laparoscopic salpingo-oophorectomies) at least one
larger secondary trocar is necessary to remove the surgical specimen
and/or to use larger instruments such as a staple gun.

TECHNIQUES FOR OPERATIVE MICROLAPAROSCOPY UNDER LOCAL ANESTHESIA

The keys to success of operative microlaparoscopy are proper patient
selection, adequate analgesia/anesthesia, good intraoperative judgment,
and quality microinstrumentation. Using the technique of diagnostic microlaparoscopy under local anesthesia with conscious sedation described in
Chapter 6 (2,3), we infiltrate one or more suprapubic sites with 1% lidocaine
with epinephrine and sodium bicarbonate before insertion of additional
trocars.

FULGURATION OF ENDOMETRIOSIS

Once the sites of endometriosis are identified, 1% plain lidocaine is applied
to the area using the suction/aspiration cannula (Fig. 8.2; see also Fig. 3.4,
B). Small superficial endometriosis implants <5 mm in diameter can be
easily fulgurated with electrosurgery (Figs. 8.3 and 8.4). I have noted that

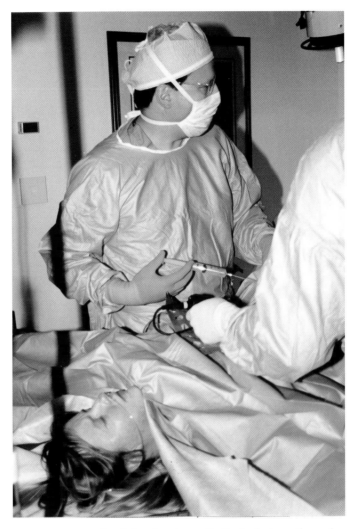

FIGURE 8.2. Applying local anesthetic to lesions through a 2-mm cannula.

the lidocaine is readily absorbed (without injecting) into the peritoneal surface and better pain relief is achieved when the lidocaine is suctioned and re-applied to the area at least four times using the cannula. With deeper lesions, injection using the needle cannula may be necessary (see Fig. 3.4, **C**). At this time biopsies can be obtained for histologic diagnosis and the implants fulgurated using the 2-mm cautery scissors at a power setting of 30 W monopolar pinpoint coagulation. Deep implants should be excised to avoid inadequate resection. This can be done with good patient comfort using deeper sedation with the sedative hypnotic propofol. Severe endometriosis *should not* be managed using this technique, because there may be increased patient discomfort and a higher risk of bleeding or other complications. A maximum surgical effort and maximum surgical result can be

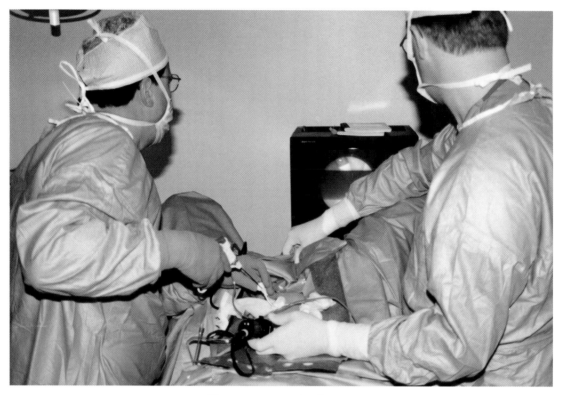

FIGURE 8.3. Electrosurgery using 2-mm cautery scissors.

realized with this technique for stage I and II endometrioses. For maximum surgical effort and maximum surgical result for stage III and IV endometrioses, operative microlaparoscopy should be done under general anesthesia because of the more extensive adhesions and deeper lesions.

LYSIS OF ADHESIONS

Pelvic adhesions have been associated with pelvic pain and infertility. As noted in Chapter 7, significant adhesions have been identified as the source of pelvic pain in some patients using the technique of conscious pain mapping (2). Studies have shown significant pain relief after laparoscopic lysis of adhesions (6,7). Primary lysis of adhesions can be achieved using the same technique of applying 1% plain lidocaine over the adhesions. Filmy adhesions are lysed without cautery using 2-mm scissors (Fig. 8.5; see also Fig. 3.5, **D**).

Thick adhesive bands should be cauterized using the 2-mm monopolar coagulation scissors at a setting of 40 W spray coagulation or the 2-mm biopolar forceps proximally and distally to prevent hemorrhage before excision (Fig. 8.6; see also Fig. 3.6, **B**). After lysis of adhesions, prophylactic prevention of postoperative adhesions can be attempted with lactated Ringer's solution (8,9).

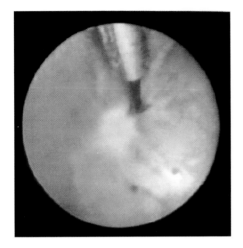

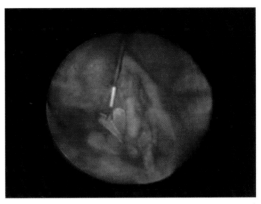

FIGURE 8.4. Fulgurating endometriosis implants using 2-mm cautery scissors.

FIGURE 8.5. Lysis of filmy adhesions using 2-mm cautery scissors.

LUNA

Women with dysmenorrhea and central uterine pain may benefit from a LUNA. Destroying the afferent sensory nerve fibers in the uterosacral ligaments provide varying degrees of pain relief (10–12). Although LUNA is not as efficacious as presacral neurectomy (12), it is a more minimally invasive procedure and can be performed under local anesthesia (2,3). After applying 1% plain lidocaine over the uterosacral ligaments several times to allow absorption of the local anesthetic, the ligaments are completely transected at their insertion into the cervix using the monopolar 2-mm cautery scissors (Fig. 8.7). When the application of lidocaine is insufficient, the drug

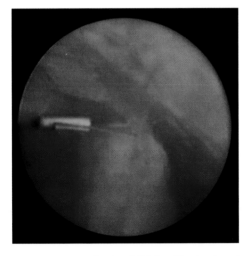

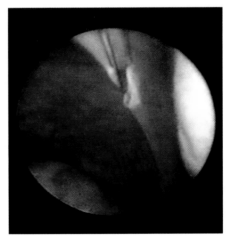

FIGURE 8.6. Lysis of thick adhesive band using 2-mm cautery scissors.

FIGURE 8.7. Microlaparoscopic LUNA procedure.

may be injected with the needle cannula; 30 W pinpoint coagulation is adequate. Although the procedure is safe, meticulous surgical technique is necessary to avoid injury to the ureters and uterine vessels.

TUBAL STERILIZATION

Laparoscopic tubal sterilization is the most frequently employed procedure for interval sterilization in the United States. The surgical and anesthetic methods used are varied. General anesthesia is the most common anesthetic method used for female sterilization procedures. Unfortunately, complications from general anesthesia are the leading cause of morbidity and mortality attributable to sterilization in the United States (13). Therefore, unless contraindicated, elective tubal sterilization procedures should be performed under local anesthesia with conscious sedation. Some authors have reported large series of tubal sterilization under local anesthesia without any increase in morbidity and mortality (14–16). Several minimally invasive microlaparoscopic techniques are available for tubal sterilization, which are described below.

BIPOLAR COAGULATION   With the recent introduction of 2-mm bipolar forceps, the coagulation method of sterilization can be performed with microinstrumentation. After insertion of a 2-mm cannula in the suprapubic region, 1% plain lidocaine is applied over the entire fallopian tubes several times. Once the tubes can be grasped and elevated without great discomfort to the patient, at least *three* contiguous areas on the tube are coagulated for a minimum of 5s, starting approximately 3 cm from the tubal insertion on the uterus. Inadequate coagulation of the tubes can result in recanalization with an increased risk of ectopic or intrauterine pregnancy. I recommend a setting of 40 W spray coagulation. The downside to this method is that surgical reversal is more difficult because about 3 cm of each fallopian tube will be destroyed.

MODIFIED POMEROY   The modified Pomeroy method is based on the same principle as the silastic band technique. Traditionally, the Pomeroy technique has been performed by removing a tube segment. The removal of the tube segment is not necessary for the success of the procedure, as demonstrated with the efficacy of the silastic band technique. The procedure can be performed with 2-mm microinstrumentation. Two suprapubic 2-mm cannulas are introduced. After advancing a grasping forceps through one of the cannulas and passing it through the Endoloop, a tubal segment is grasped and the Endoloop placed over the segment and fastened. The suture is then cut using 2-mm noncautery scissors.

CLIP METHOD (HULKA CLIP OR FILSHIE CLIP)   I use the clip method for tubal sterilization in an awake patient for several reasons. It is the fastest

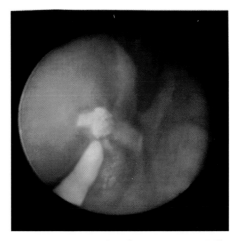

FIGURE 8.8. Microlaparoscopic Hulka
clip tubal sterilization.

to perform, produces the least amount of discomfort to the patient (because
it does not bunch up the tissue), and is bloodless. In addition, it has the
greatest chance for surgical tubal anastomosis, because only a small segment of each fallopian tube is destroyed (Fig. 8.8). The only disadvantage
of this technique is that microinstrumentation cannot be used exclusively,
because a 7-mm trocar is required in the suprapubic area to introduce the
clip applicator. After infiltration with local anesthesia over the desired
suprapubic region, a 7-mm trocar is inserted, and 1% plain lidocaine is
applied over the fallopian tubes. After the clip (Hulka or Filshie) is loaded
on the clip applicator and advanced through the trocar, the clip is applied
perpendicular to the long axis of the fallopian tube at the level of the midis-
thmus. The site of the 7-mm trocar can then be closed with a subcuticular
stitch of 4-0 Vicryl.

OVARIAN DRILLING

Ovarian drilling is a minimally invasive technique for the surgical management of polycystic ovarian syndrome; it is extensively described in Chapter 12.

MICROLAPAROSCOPIC APPENDECTOMY
UNDER LOCAL ANESTHESIA

The appendix is an underappreciated source of pain in women with chronic
pelvic pain. Incidental appendectomy has been advocated in patients with
chronic pelvic pain who are undergoing abdominal surgery (17–19). Limitations in the evaluation of the appendix under general anesthesia result
from the lack of intraoperative patient feedback. Although the potential

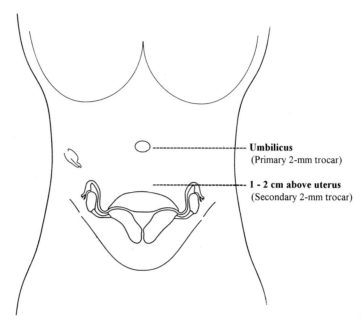

Umbilicus
(Primary 2-mm trocar)

1 - 2 cm above uterus
(Secondary 2-mm trocar)

FIGURE 8.9. Trocar placements for conscious pain mapping of the appendix.

yield of appendiceal disease associated with the grossly normal appendix has been demonstrated, a higher percentage yield has been reported when the appendix is evaluated using conscious pain mapping (2, 20).

Laparoscopic appendectomy under general anesthesia has been extensively described, primarily in the general surgery literature. I have found it useful to develop a minimally invasive microlaparoscopic technique for appendectomy that, in selected patients, can be performed under local anesthesia (21).

After conducting conscious pain mapping (Chapter 7), if the appendix is inordinately tender or appears to be anatomically distorted (i.e., fecalith), the midline suprapubic 2-mm trocar is removed and re-inserted over the right lower quadrant after infiltration with local anesthesia. The previous suprapubic incision from which the 2-mm trocar was removed is further infiltrated with local anesthesia, and the incision is extended to the left to accommodate a 12-mm trocar (Figs. 8.9 and 8.10). The appendix and mesoappendix are irrigated with 1% plain lidocaine. All appendiceal adhesions are lysed with the 2-mm cautery scissors. The appendix is then grasped and linearized with 2-mm grasping forceps. Using a Multifire ENDO GIA 30 stapler (U.S. Surgical Corp., Norwalk, CT), the surgeon divides the mesoappendix. This dissection is continued to the appendiceal-cecal junction. If the appendiceal artery is not contained within the staples, hemostasis can be achieved with the 2-mm bipolar forceps. Once the appendix is isolated, the stapler is placed at the base of the appendix, where the appendix is separated from the cecum (Fig. 8.11). The appendix is then removed through the 12-mm trocar.

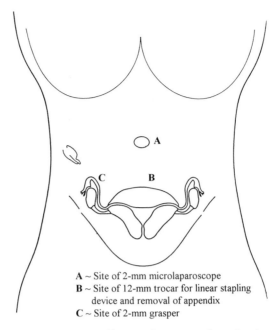

A ~ Site of 2-mm microlaparoscope
B ~ Site of 12-mm trocar for linear stapling
    device and removal of appendix
C ~ Site of 2-mm grasper

FIGURE 8.10. Trocar placements for microlaparoscopic appendectomy.

After irrigation with saline, the only trocar site that requires suturing is the 12-mm one. In selected patients who have undergone their appendectomy under local anesthesia with conscious sedation, the procedure has been completed with good patient comfort. In some cases, the patient has required more fentanyl, in others the use of propofol. Patients who require an appendectomy and are uncomfortable after conscious pain mapping or operative microlaparoscopy under local anesthesia can still benefit from

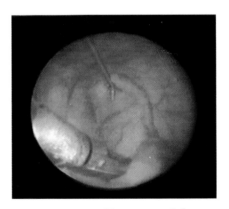

FIGURE 8.11. Placement of the staple gun on the appendix.

this minimally invasive technique for appendectomy under general anesthesia.

MINIMIZING SURGICAL RISK IN PATIENTS WITH PREVIOUS MULTIPLE SURGERIES

In the 1990s, many procedures previously routinely done under laparotomy were performed with laparoscopy. This is especially true for women with previous multiple pelvic and abdominal surgeries. With the availability of microlaparoscopy today, the once-novel larger Hasson cannula has been replaced with the 2-mm Veress needle and cannula in these high-risk patients (22). The Hasson cannula was developed to reduce the risk of blind entry into the peritoneal cavity. Injury to the bowel, however, has been reported to occur at the same rate as blind entry with this technique (23). Unrecognized bowel injury during laparoscopy is very rare. Recognized accidental bowel perforations occur in < 1% of laparoscopic procedures (24). Unfortunately, complications can and do occur even with the experienced laparoscopist. Current data on laparoscopic complications are based on case reports and small series (25). Bowel perforations from 2-mm instrumentation can be managed conservatively without suturing, provided that the site of injury is not actively leaking stool or bleeding. An added advantage of microlaparoscopy is that the microlaparoscope can be inserted immediately without removing the cannula in situations when perforation is suspected. When the site of perforation is free of adhesions and in need of repair, the bowel can be sutured externally by withdrawing it through a 12-mm trocar (26).

REFERENCES

1. Fervers C. Die Laparoskopie mit dem cystoskop: ein beitrag zur vereinfachung der technik und zur endoskopischen Strangdurtrennung in der Bauchhohle. Med Klin 29:1042–1045, 1933.

2. Almeida OD Jr , Val-Gallas JM. Conscious pain mapping. J Am Assoc Gynecol Laparosc 4:587–590, 1997.

3. Almeida OD Jr, Val-Gallas JM. A protocol for conscious sedation in microlaparoscopy. J Am Assoc Gynecol Laparosc 4:591–594, 1997.

4. Almeida OD Jr, Val-Gallas JM, Rizk B. Appendectomy under local anaesthesia following conscious pain mapping with microlaparoscopy. Hum Reprod 13:588–590, 1998.

5. Almeida OD Jr, Rizk B. Microlaparoscopic ovarian drilling under local anesthesia. Middle East Fertil Soc J 3:189–191, 1998.

6. Steege JF, Stout AL. Resolution of chronic pelvic pain after laparoscopic lysis of adhesions Am J Obstet Gynecol 165:278–281, 1991.

7. Sutton C, MacDonald R. Laser laparoscopic adhesiolysis. J Gynecol Surg 6:155, 1990.

8. Tulandi T, Murray C, Guralnick M. Adhesion formation and reproductive outcome after myomectomy and second-look laparoscopy. Obstet Gynecol 82:213–215, 1993.

9. Pagidas K, Tulandi T. Effects of Ringer's lactate, Interceed (TC7) and Gore-Tex surgical membrane on postsurgical adhesion formation. Fertil Steril 57:199–201, 1992.

10. Chen FP, Chang SD, Chu KK, Soong YK. Comparison of laparoscopic presacral neurectomy and laparoscopic uterine nerve ablation for primary dysmenorrhea. J Reprod Med 41:463–466, 1996.

11. Lichten EM, Bombard J. Surgical treatment of dysmenorrhea with laparoscopic uterine nerve ablation. J Reprod Med 32:37–41, 1987.

12. Damaro MA, Horowitz IR, Rock JA. The role of uterosacral ligament resection in conservative operations for recurrent endometriosis. J Gynecol Surg 10:57–61, 1994.

13. Peterson HB, SeStefano F, Rubin GL, et al. Deaths attributable to tubal sterilization in the United States, 1977 to 1981. Am J Obstet Gynecol. 146:131–136, 1983.

14. Wheeles CR Jr. Outpatient laparoscopic sterilization under local anesthesia. Obstet Gynecol 39:767–770, 1972.

15. Penfield AJ. Twenty-two years of office and outpatient laparoscopy: current techniques and why I chose them. J Am Assoc Gynecol Laparosc 2:365–368, 1995.

16. Metha PV. A total of 250,136 laparoscopic sterilizations by a single operator. Br J Obstet Gynaecol 96:1024–1034, 1989.

17. Fischer LC. Could the appendix be removed in all cases where the abdomen is opened for other causes? Atlanta J Rec Med 10:410–414, 1909.

18. Goldspohn A. Why the vermiform appendix should usually be removed when an abdominal incision made for other causes is available and the condition of the patient admits of the additional operating. Ill Med J 19:593–603, 1911.

19. Fisher KS, Ross DS. Guidelines for therapeutic decision in incidental appendectomy. Surg Gynecol Obstet 171:95–98, 1990.

20. Almeida OD Jr, Val-Gallas JM. Conscious pain mapping of the appendix with microlaparoscopy for the evaluation of women with chronic pelvic pain. Middle East Fertil Soc J, in press.

21. Almeida OD Jr, Val-Gallas JM, Rizk B. Appendectomy under local anaesthesia following conscious pain mapping with microlaparoscopy. Hum Reprod 13:588–590, 1998.

22. Hasson HM. Open laparoscopy: a report of 150 cases. J Reprod Med 12:234–238, 1974.

23. Yuzpe AA. Pneumoperitoneum needle and trocar injuries in laparoscopy. J Reprod Med 35:485–490, 1990.

24. Minoli G, Terruazzi V, Tadeo G. Laparoscopy: the question of proper gas. Gastrointest Endosc 29:325, 1983.

25. Almeida OD Jr, Val-Gallas JM. Small trocar perforation of the small bowel: a case report. J Soc Laparoendosc Surg 2:289–290, 1998.

26. Laparoscopic management of complications. In Hulka JF, Reich H, eds. Textbook of laparoscopy. Philadelphia Saunders, 1998: 516–517.

Office Microlaparoscopy

Oscar D. Almeida, Jr., M.D., F.A.C.O.G., F.A.C.S.

Minimally invasive surgery continues to revolutionize and redefine office gynecology. Outdated procedures once done in the traditional hospital operating room under general anesthesia such as laser conization of the cervix for cervical intraepithelial neoplasia (CIN) have given way to the less invasive loop electrosurgical excision procedure(LEEP) of the cervix under local anesthesia performed in the physician's office. Gynecologists, patients and third-party payers have realized the benefits of doing surgical procedures in the office setting. One of the most significant recent events in this evolution has been the introduction of office microlaparoscopy under local anesthesia, for both diagnostic and advanced operative procedures. Some of these advantages are summarized in Table 9.1.

TABLE 9.1. BENEFITS OF PERFORMING OFFICE MICROLAPAROSCOPY
UNDER LOCAL ANESTHESIA

- Cost containment
- Less paperwork (unnecessary duplication of information and record keeping)
- Easier scheduling (for both physician and patient)
- No waiting for other surgeons to finish their operations/elimination of travel time
- Conscious patient is helpful in making diagnosis
- Recovery time is shorter (faster return to work and normal activities)
- Procedure is more minimally invasive
- Less costly to insurance carrier in terms of dollars compared to hospital procedures under general anesthesia

Microlaparoscopy, Edited by Oscar D. Almeida Jr.
ISBN 0-471-34574-1 Copyright © 2000 by Wiley-Liss, Inc.

Office microlaparoscopy has evolved primarily from the methods previously established for outpatient office laparoscopic tubal ligation (1–3). The purpose of doing office microlaparoscopy under local anesthesia with conscious sedation is to perform diagnostic and therapeutic manuevers in a minimally invasive manner in selected patients. In the 1997 American Association of Gynecologic Laparoscopists membership survey; "Practice Profiles," 73 respondents perform office laparoscopy and 135 do microlaparoscopy under local anesthesia (4). When asked which laparoscopic procedures were appropriate for the office setting, 51% stated sterilization; 37%, second-look laparoscopy; and 17%, postoperative lysis of adhesions. My general sense of the applicability of this surgical approach is that many women who undergo traditional laparoscopic surgery under general anesthesia in the hospital or ambulatory surgery center can have their procedures done less invasively in the physician's office.

Until recently, most reported office microlaparoscopic procedures have been diagnostic in nature (5,6). Novel advances in technique and instrumentation have unlocked the door for several operative microlaparoscopic procedures to be performed in the office under local anesthesia with conscious sedation. These include electrosurgery to fulgurate endometriosis, primary lysis of adhesions, and LUNA in patients with chronic pelvic pain (7–10). No deep side wall dissections or fulguration of endometriosis near the ureters or blood vessels should be done, to avoid complications. Female sterilization as described in Chapter 8, second-look microlaparoscopy, and infertility evaluations can easily be performed in the office setting.

The question of safety while performing both diagnostic and operative microlaparoscopy under local anesthesia in an office-based, free-standing facility outside of the hospital or outpatient surgery center presents legitimate concerns. Procedures done at all three sites must provide equal patient safety. Strict adherence to protocols for patient selection, surgical technique, and patient monitoring is essential (9). At all times, a *minimum* of two ACLS-certified gynecologists and an ACLS-certified registered nurse must be present during office microlaparoscopic procedures to have the personnel necessary to handle an emergency. A crash cart containing resuscitative and reversal agents, in addition to a defibrillator *must* be readily available. An emergency plan containing a plan of action, emergency telephone numbers, and protocols for patient transport and hospital admission should be in place. Patient monitoring is accomplished by continuous pulse oximeter, electrocardiogram, and respiration and temperature evaluation. Blood pressure is measured every 3 min. We use the multifunction Datascope monitor (Paramus, NJ) in our office laparoscopy suite.

Patient selection for office procedures is crucial. Many patients who can have their procedures successfully performed under local anesthesia with conscious sedation in a hospital or ambulatory center may not be good candidates for an office procedure; because, for example, the unavailability of

TABLE 9.2. CONTRAINDICATIONS TO OFFICE MICROLAPAROSCOPIC
PROCEDURES

- History of psychiatric anxiety disorders
- Morbid obesity (relative contraindication)
- History of intolerance to benzodiazepines or lidocaine
- Long-term drug addiction
- Cardiac or respiratory disease
- Neuropathic or swallowing disorders
- Hepatic or renal encephalopathy
- Multiple previous pelvic/abdominal surgeries (relative contraindication)
- Patients anticipated to require a more extensive surgical procedure under general anesthesia

general anesthesia and/or the inability to perform more complex operative microlaparoscopic procedures in the office setting. In addition, some patients with complex medical problems should be monitored by an anesthesiologist. Selected women for the office procedures include preoperative ASA physical status level 1 or 2 as documented by history, physical examination, and thorough laboratory testing. Preoperative laboratory tests include CBC, electrolytes, liver function tests, urinalysis, hCG, ECG and chest x-ray. Table 9.2 summarizes contraindications for office procedures. Patients not meeting selection criteria should have their surgery performed in a hospital or ambulatory surgery center, where they can be monitored by an anesthesiologist. Women anticipated to have worse than stage II endometriosis should have their procedure done under general anesthesia.

After fasting for a minimum of 7 h before surgery, an intravenous line is started and the patient receives a 500 mL preload of lactated Ringer's solution. Conscious sedation is administered per our protocol (atropine 0.2 mg, ondansetron hydrochloride 4 mg, midazolam hydrochloride 2 mg, and fentanyl citrate 250 μg titrated to effect) by one of the gynecologists until satisfactory levels of sedation and comfort are obtained and monitoring parameters achieved (Fig. 9.1) (8). After this, the registered nurse continues monitoring the patient, charting data every 5 min as done since arrival into the operating room and further titrating the medications as instructed by the physicians.

The patient is sterily prepared and draped, and a Foley catheter inserted. Paracervical, periumbilical, and suprapubic blocks are administered at the operative sites with 10 mL of 1% lidocaine with epinephrine 1:100,000

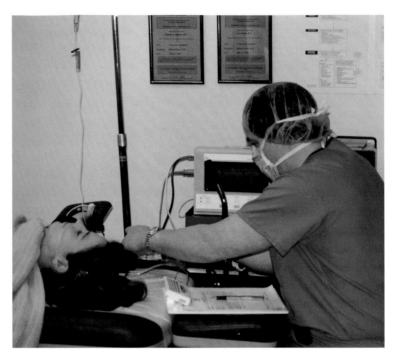

FIGURE 9.1. Conscious sedation being administered by an ACLS-certified gynecologist.

buffered with sodium bicarbonate (10:1 dilution). Diagnostic and operative microlaparoscopy can then be performed. It cannot be overemphasized that the microlaparoscopic instrumentation, including the microlaparoscope, light cable and light source, insufflator and tubing, and video camera and television should be set up and tested for proper function before the patient has her intravenous line started.

Office microlaparoscopy facility considerations include room size, temperature control mechanism, electrical outlet support, lighting, scrub sink, and nearby restroom. Careful planning must include the proper facility, equipment, and supplies needed in the event of urgent and emergent situations. (Fig. 9.2 and 9.3).

The primary limitation of office microlaparoscopy is that if more extensive surgery is necessary, the office facility and setup may not be able to accommodate it. Although we have performed microlaparoscopic appendectomies under local anesthesia with conscious sedation (10), complex operative procedures such as this should be done in a hospital or ambulatory surgery center. To date, all patients have tolerated their office diagnostic (including conscious pain mapping) and operative procedures when we have followed our strict protocol for patient selection, conscious sedation, and microlaparoscopic technique. None of the patients has required intubation, bagging by mask, had an oxygen saturation (SaO_2) below 94% or

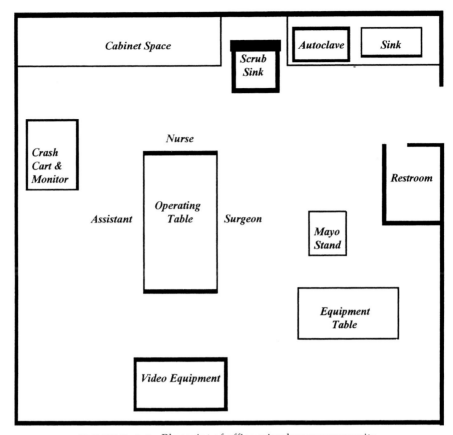

FIGURE 9.2. Blueprint of office microlaparoscopy suite.

required the use of reversal agents. No patient has experienced hypotension, tachycardia, nausea, vomiting, or dyspnea or has required being seen by either the surgeon or their family physician before their scheduled 2 week post-operative visit due to severe pain or other complications. No patient has required hospitalization. No transfusion of blood or blood products has been required in any case. All patients have walked out of the office unassisted within 1 h after completion of surgery.

A current obstacle frequently encountered with office laparoscopy is the lack of insurance coverage. Laparoscopic procedures done under local anesthesia with conscious sedation are more cost-effective than is hospital-based traditional laparoscopy under general anesthesia (5,6,11,12). One study (6) evaluated the costs of office microlaparoscopy and reported an almost 80% reduction in billed charges. At this time, only a few insurance carriers reimburse fees for office laparoscopy. This should change in the near future as more physicians and insurance carriers embrace the concept of minimally invasive surgery.

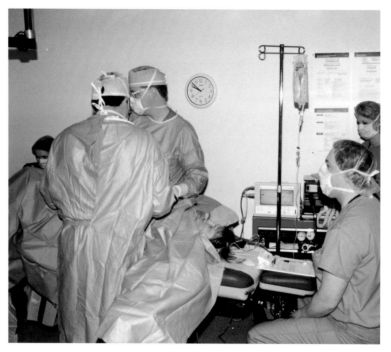

FIGURE 9.3. Office microlaparoscopy procedure.

REFERENCES

1. Wheeless C Jr. Outpatient laparoscopic sterilization under local anesthesia. Obstet Gynecol 39:767–770, 1972.

2. Penfield AJ. Laparoscopic sterilization under local anesthesia. Obstet Gynecol 12:251–253, 1974.

3. Love BR, McCorvey R, McCorvey M. Low-cost office laparoscopic sterilization. J Am Assoc Gynecol Laparosc 4:379–382, 1994.

4. Hulka JF, Levy BS, Luciano AA, Parker WH, Phillips JM. 1977 AAGL membership survey: practice profiles. J Am Assoc Gynecol Laparosc. 5:93–96, 1998.

5. Feste JR. Use of optical catheters for diagnostic office laparoscopy. J Reprod Med 41:307–312, 1996.

6. Palter SF, Olive DL. Office microlaparoscopy under local anesthesia for chronic pelvic pain. J Am Assoc Gynecol Laparosc 3:359–364, 1996.

7. Almeida OD Jr, Val-Gallas JM. Conscious pain mapping. J Am Assoc Gynecol Laparosc 4:587–590, 1997.

8. Almeida OD Jr, Val-Gallas JM, Browning JL. A protocol for conscious sedation in microlaparoscopy. J Am Assoc Gynecol Laparosc 4:591–594, 1997.

9. Almeida OD Jr, Val-Gallas JM. Office microlaparoscopy under local anesthesia in the diagnosis and treatment of chronic pelvic pain. J Am Assoc Gynecol Laparosc 5:407–410,1998.

10. Steege JF. Repeated clinic laparoscopy for the treatment of pelvic adhesions: a pilot study. Obstet Gynecol 83:276–279, 1994.

11. Almeida OD Jr, Val-Gallas JM, Rizk B. Appendectomy under local anaesthesia following conscious pain mapping with microlaparoscopy. Hum Reprod. 13:588–590, 1998.

12. Squires RH, Morriss G, Schlueterman S, et al. Efficacy, safety and cost of intravenous sedation versus general anesthesia in children undergoing endoscopic procedures. Gastrointest Endosc 41:99–104, 1995.

MICROLAPAROSCOPY IN EVALUATION OF THE INFERTILE PATIENT

BOTROS RIZK, M.D., M.A., M.R.C.O.G., F.R.C.S.(C.), H.C.L.D., F.A.C.O.G., F.A.C.S.

The use of laparoscopy for infertility was pioneered by Palmer in France and Steptoe in England in the mid-twentieth century. Their contribution to our field is monumental and will have repercussions for years to come. Today laparoscopy is part of the standard management of all infertility treatment and is incorporated in some forms of ART.

The advances in microlaparoscopy during the last several years have been outstanding. The improvement in illumination and visualization in these miniaturized endoscopes have made it possible to diagnose and treat different forms of pelvic infertility. In this chapter, I review the role of microlaparoscopy in the management of infertility.

MICROLAPAROSCOPY IN THE EVALUATION OF THE PELVIS

The place of laparoscopy as a first-line infertility investigation has waxed and waned over the years. In couples presenting with primary infertility, the evaluation of semen parameters and ovulation presents the first investigative step before proceeding to diagnostic laparoscopy. It is, therefore, reasonable in some cases to consider ovulation induction with clomiphene citrate before endoscopic evaluation. Microlaparoscopy encompasses the next phase of evaluation in patients who have failed 3 months of medical management. This survey of the pelvis is carefully conducted to identify pelvic endometriosis, and peritubal and periovarian adhesions. The fimbriae is evaluated for the presence of phimosis or occlusion. Chromotubation can be easily performed (Fig. 10.1). The evaluation of the pelvis using

Microlaparoscopy, Edited by Oscar D. Almeida Jr.
ISBN 0-471-34574-1 Copyright © 2000 by Wiley-Liss, Inc.

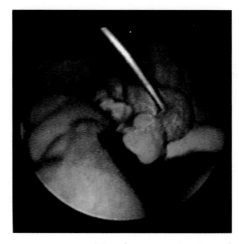

FIGURE 10.1. Microlaparoscopic view of
the fallopian tube during chromotubation.

microlaparoscopy could be performed in an office laparoscopy suite,
outpatient ambulatory surgery center, or traditional hospital operating
room.

SALPINGOSTOMY AND FIMBRIOPLASTY USING MICROLAPAROSCOPY

In 1977, Gomel (1) reported four pregnancies in nine women undergoing laparoscopic salpingostomy. Today laparoscopic salpingostomies are
routinely performed (Tables 10.1 and 10.2). With the advancement
of microsurgical instrumentation, fimbrioplasty and salpingostomy can
be performed using a 2-mm cautery scissors and bipolar electrosurgical
coagulator.

TABLE.10.1. PREGNANCY OUTCOME OF SALPINGOSTOMY BY LAPAROSCOPY

Number	% Pregnancy	% Intrauterine Pregnancy	% Ectopic	Reference
9	—	44.4	0	1
38	26	—	—	2
19	10	—	10	3
21	24	19	5	4
55	20	—	15	5
87		33.3	6.9	6
22	22.7	—	?	7
42	35.7	—	15.4	8
81	37	32.1	4.9	9

TABLE 10.2. FIMBRIOPLASTY BY LAPARASOPY: FERTILITY RESULTS

Number	Intrauterine Pregnancy		Ectopic Pregnancy		Reference
	n	%	n	%	
40	20	50	2	5	10
31	8	25.8	4	12.9	11
71	28	39.4	6	8.5	

MICROLAPAROSCOPY IN THE PREPARATION FOR ART

Microlaparoscopy is a useful tool in the evaluation of patients considering assisted reproductive technology. In 1976, Steptoe and Edwards (12) published the first pregnancy resulting from in vitro fertilization (IVF) (12). Unfortunately, it resulted in an ectopic pregnancy. This led Steptoe to recommend laparoscopic tubal occlusion before IVF (13). Two decades later, laparoscopic tubal occlusion is not practiced anymore for the following reasons. First, tubal occlusion does not prevent interstitial pregnancies. Bowel adhesions to the diathermized fallopian tubes interfere with future laparoscopic oocyte recoveries, which was practiced in the early 1980s. In addition, a small portion of patients with tubal disease would spontaneously conceive.

The situation went full circle in the 1990s. Before the era of intracytoplasmic sperm injection (ICSI), Rizk and colleagues (14) compared the fertilization and implantation rates in different categories of patients considering IVF between 1985 and 1989. The fertilization rate was highest in patients undergoing IVF for tubal disease and lowest in couples with male factor infertility. The implantation rate, however, was highest in couples

TABLE 10.3. COMPARISION OF PREGNANCY RATES AFTER IVF IN PATIENTS WITH AND WITHOUT HYDROSALPINGES

Pregnancy Rate/ Embryo Transfer (%)		Delivery Rate/ Embryo Transfer (%)		Reference
Hydrosalpinx	Control Group	Hydrosalpinx	Control Group	
13	26	7	18	15
10	30	7	21	16
18	31	10	25	17
10	23	10	21	18
17	37	—	—	19
39	45	—	—	20
25	33	—	—	21
3	42	8	39	22

TABLE 10.4. EMBRYONIC IMPLANTATION RATES IN THE PRESENCE OF
HYDROSALPINGES

Hydrosalpinx (%)	Control Group (%)	Reference
3	10	16
8	12	17
4	10	23
4	11	18
10	13	20
3	16	22

with male infertility and lowest in couples with tubal disease. Although this study analyzed 3,505 IVF cycles and > 21,000 oocytes, there was no statistical difference between the different groups of patients. This highlights the possibility of a negative effect of tubal factor infertility on the implantation rate. The effect of a hydrosalpinx in particular would have been very interesting to analyze separately.

Several publications have addressed the effect of tubal disease with and without hydrosalpinges on the pregnancy and implantation rates in IVF (Tables 10.3 and 10.4). In all studies, the hydrosalpinges appeared to have a negative effect on the implantation and pregnancy rates, and in some studies the difference was statistically significant. These results have led some clinicians to recommend laparoscopic salpingectomies before IVF in patients with hydrosalpinges. This clinical situation should be individualized, and it is anticipated that microlaparoscopy will play a major role in the evaluation of selected cases.

MICROSURGICAL LAPAROSCOPIC TUBAL ANASTOMOSIS

Swolin (24) has led the way for the advancement of microsurgical techniques for infertility surgery. He proposed the use of magnification and delicate instrumentation for adhesiolysis and neosalpingostomy. Winston (25) and Gomel (1) separately published their series of microsurgical reversal of sterilization. Since then microsurgical techniques have become the gold standard for tubal anastomosis. Koh (26) refined the techniques of laparoscopic tubal anastomosis and analyzed the clinical results in a systematic way. The absence of stereoscopic vision is initially troublesome; however, adaptation occurs rapidly. The closed environment and use of a pneumoperitoneum to obtain exposure without packing might be beneficial in reduction of adhesion formation.

Koh and Janik (27) achieved a cumulative pregnancy rate of 35.5, 54.8, 67.7, and 71% at 1, 3, 6, and 12 months, respectively. The surgical duration in the first 10 cases decreased from a mean of 5.9 h for the first 5 cases to 3.1

h for the second 5 cases. Currently, the operating time ranges from 1 to 2 h
(26). In 1998, Almeida and Rizk (28) anticipated the use of microlaparoscopy for tubal anastomosis; ongoing research to evaluate the feasibility of this technique continues. The authors (29) reviewed the European and
American experience and concluded that in selected cases microlaparoscopy is the way for the future in the area of tubal anastomosis.

MICROLAPAROSCOPY IN THE MANAGEMENT OF HETEROTOPIC PREGNANCIES

Heterotopic pregnancy is seen in 1% of all pregnancies after ART (30). The
management of these pregnancies is challenging because of the presence of
the concomitant intrauterine pregnancy. Methotrexate cannot be employed
for the treatment of the ectopic pregnancy, owing to the risk imposed on the
intrauterine fetus. Because microlaparoscopy minimally disturbs the intra-
abdominal milieu, it is the treatment of choice for evaluation of the
extrauterine pregnancy.

The outcome of the intrauterine pregnancy is usually successful. A
multicenter study (31) revealed that the high prevalence of tubal damage
and multiple tubal transfer are the predisposing factors to heterotopic pregnancies. Transvaginal is superior to transabdominal ultrasound in diagnosing the extrauterine pregnancies and should be performed (Table 10.5). The
presence of an intrauterine gestational sac in a patient without symptoms
should not exclude the diagnosis of a concomitant extrauterine pregnancy
until the pelvis has been carefully visualized. Rarely, bilateral tubal pregnancies occur after assisted conception (32). Early diagnosis of ectopic pregnancies before rupture prevents mortality, reduces morbidity, and offers the
chance of selecting patients for conservative treatment. Microlaparoscopic
salpingectomy can easily be performed before the rupture of the ectopic
pregnancy.

THE ROLE OF MICROLAPAROSCOPY IN THE PREVENTION OF OVARIAN HYPERSTIMULATION SYNDROME IN PATIENTS WITH POLYCYSTIC OVARIAN SYNDROME

Ovarian hyperstimulation syndrome (OHSS) is the most serious complication of ovulation induction (33). OHSS has been recently reclassified into
moderate and severe (34). PCOS has been identified as the predisposing factor for OHSS in the majority of patients (35). In 1991 Rizk and Aboulghar
outlined the prevention and management of OHSS (36). In 1999, Abdalla
and Rizk (29) devised an algorithm for the management of PCOS. They em-
phasized the role of a low-dose step-up protocol of gonadotropins for the
prevention of OHSS. The long protocol of hypothalamic-pituitary ovarian
downregulation using a combination of gonadotropin-releasing hormone

TABLE 10.5. USE OF SONOGRAPHY IN THE DIAGNOSIS OF INTRAUTERINE AND EXTRAUTERINE PREGNANCIES.[a]

Patient Number	Clinical Presentation	Diagnosis	Gestational Sacs in Utero	Ectopic Pregnancy	Fetal Hearts in Utero	Intrauterine Pregnancy	Duration of Pregnancy at Time of Diagnosis (weeks)
1	Abdominal pain	Abdominal	1	1	1	6	8
2	Abdominal pain	Abdominal	3	2	0	6	0
3	Abdominal pain	Abdominal	1	0	0	5	0
4	Abdominal pain	Abdominal	1	0	1	6	6
5	Abdominal pain	Abdominal	1	0	0	5	0
6	Abdominal pain	Abdominal	1	0	1	7	7
7	Abdominal pain, bleeding	Abdominal	2	1	1	7	7
8	Abdominal pain, bleeding	Abdominal	1	0	0	7	0
9	Abdominal pain, bleeding	Abdominal	1	0	1	8	8
10	Acute abdomen	Abdominal	1	0	0	5	0
11	Acute abdomen	Abdominal	2	2	0	8	0
12	No symptoms	Abdominal	1	1	0	6	0
13	No symptoms	Abdominal plus bleeding	1	1	1	7	7
14	No symptoms	Abdominal plus bleeding	2	2	1	7	7
15	No symptoms	Abdominal plus bleeding	1	1	1	7	7
16	No symptoms	Abdominal plus bleeding	1	1	1	7	7
17	No symptoms	Abdominal plus bleeding	1	1	1	7	7

[a]Adapted from Rizk et al. (30).

agonist and recombinant gonadotropins is successful but carries a high risk of OHSS. Electrosurgical diathermy has been proposed as the treatment of choice for reducing the possibility of OHSS (37). Microlaparoscopy offers the ability to perform ovarian drilling in a minimally invasive fashion (38). Using microinstrumentation in these high-risk patients may offer the possibility of reducing ovarian trauma and pelvic adhesions.

In summary, microlaparoscopy is particularly suitable in the evaluation of the pelvis of infertile patients. In addition, it can be tailored to prepare the pelvis for ART in patients who are candidates for this treatment modality. Microlaparoscopic salpingectomies can be performed for hydrosalpinges when the tubes are unsalvageable. These advances in microlaparoscopy show great promise for the field of infertility.

REFERENCES

1. Gomel V. Tubal reconstruction by microsurgery. Fertil Steril 28:59, 1977.

2. Mettler L, Giesel H, Semm K. Treatment of female infertility due to tubal obstruction by operative laparoscopy. Fertil Steril 32:384–388, 1979.

3. Fayez JA. An assessment of the role of operative laparoscopy in tuboplasty. Fertil Steril 39:476–479, 1983.

4. Daniell JF, Herbert CM. Laparoscopic salpingostomy utilizing the CO_2 laser. Fertil Steril 41:558–563, 1984.

5. Audebert A, Hedon B, Arnal F et al. Therapeutic strategies in tubal infertility with distal pathology. Hum Repro 6:1439–1442, 1991.

6. Canis M, Mage G, Pouly Jl et al. Laparoscopic distal tuboplasty: report of 87 cases and a four year experience. Fertil Steril 56:616–621, 1991.

7. McComb P, Paleologou A. The intussusception salpingostomy technique for the therapy of distal oviductual occlusion at laparoscopy. Obstet Gynecol 78:443–447, 1991.

8. Dubuisson JB, Chapron C, Morice P et al. Laparoscopic salpingostomy: Fertility results according to the tubal mucosal appearance. Hum Repro 9:334–339, 1994.

9. Nezhat C, Nezhat F, Nezhat C. Operative laparoscopy (minimally invasive surgery): state of the art. J Gynecol Surg 8:111–141, 1992.

10. Gomel V. Salpingo-ovariolysis by laparoscopy in infertility. Fertil Steril 40:607–611, 1983.

11. Dubuisson JB, Bouquet de Joliniere J, Aubriot FX et al. Terminal tuboplasties by laparoscopy By laparoscopy: 65 consecutive cases. Fertil Steril 54:401–403, 1990.

12. Steptoe PC, Edwards RG. Reimplantation of a human embryo with subsequent tubal pregnancy. Lancet 1:880–882, 1976.

13. Rizk B. The outcome of assisted reproductive technology. In Brinsden P, ed., A textbook of in vitro fertilization and assisted reproduction. Carnforth, UK:Parthenon, 1999:311–332.

14. Rizk B, Davies M, Kingsland C, Mason BA. How many embryos should be replaced in an *in vitro* fertilisation programme? Paper presented at the sixth

world congress for *In Vitro* Fertilisation and Alternate Conception Techniques, Jerusalem, 1989.

15. Strandell A, Waldenstrom U, Nilsson L et al. Hydrosalpinx reduces in-vitro fertilization/embryo transfer pregnancy rates. Hum Repro 9:861–863, 1994.

16. Anderson AN, Yue Z, Meng FJ, Petersen K. Low implantation rate after in-vitro fertilization in patients with hydrosalpinges diagnoses by ultrasonography. Hum Repro 9:1935–1938, 1994.

17. Kassabji M, Sims JA, Butler L, Muasher SJ. Reduced pregnancy outcome in patients With unilateral or bilateral hydrosalpinx after in-virto fertilization. Eur J Obstet Gynecol Reprod Biol 56:129–132, 1994.

18. Katz E, Akman M, Damewood MD, Gracia JE. Deleterious effect of the presence of hydrosalpinx on implantation and pregnancy rates with in-vitro fertilization. Fertil Steril 66:122–125, 1996.

19. Blazar AS, Alexander K, Seifer DB et al. Absence of an effect of hydrosalpinx on pregnancy rate in in-vitro fertlization. In: 51st Annual Meeting of the American Fertility Society, Seattle, WA: American Society for Reproductive Medicine, 1995 (Abstract).

20. Sharara FI, Scott RT, Marut EL, Queenan JT Jr. In-vitro fertilization outcome in women with hydrosalpinx. Hum Repro 11:526–530, 1996.

21. Shelton KE, Butler L, Toner JP et al. Salpingectomy improves the pregnancy rate in in-vitro fertilization patients with hydrosalpinx. Hum Repro 11:523–525, 1996.

22. Murray DL, Sagoskin AW, Widra EA, Levy MJ. The adverse effect of hydrosalpinges on in-vitro fertilization pregnancy rates and the benefit of surgical correction. Fertil Steril 69:41–45, 1988.

23. Vandromme J. Chasse E, Lejeune B et al. Hydrosalpinges in-vitro fertilization: an unfavorable prognostic feature. Hum Repro 10:576–579, 1999.

24. Swolin K. Beitrage zur operativen Behandlung der weiblichen sterilitat: experimentelle und klinische studien, 1967.

25. Winston RML. Microsurgical tubocornual anastomosis for reversal of sterilization. Lancet 1:284, 1977.

26. Koh CH. Laparoscopic microsurgical tubal anastomosis. In Sutton C, Diamond M, eds., Endoscopic surgery for gynecologists. London:Saunders, 1998:176–185.

27. Koh CH, Janik GM. Laparoscopic microsurgical tubal anastomosis. Results of forty consecutive cases. Paper presented at the 52nd annual meeting of the American Society of Reproductive Medicine. Boston, Mass. 1996.

28. Almeida OD Jr, Rizk B. Microlaparoscopy: its evolution, present and future. Middle East Fertil Soc J 3:286–287, 1998.

29. Abdalla HI, Rizk B, (eds.), Assisted reproductive technology. Oxford, UK: Health Press,1999.

30. Rizk B, Tan SL, Morcos S, et al. Heterotopic pregnancies following *in vitro* fertilization and embryo transfer. Am J Obstet Gynecol 164:161–164, 1991.

31. Rizk B, Dimitry ES, Morcos S, et al. A multicentre study on combined intrauterine and extrauterine pregnancy after IVF. Paper presented at the second joint meeting of the European Society for Human Reproduction and Embryology, and the European Sterility Congress Organisation, Milan, Italy, 1990.

32. Rizk B, Morcos S, Avery S, et al. Rare ectopic pregnancies after *in vitro* fertilisation: one unilateral twin and four bilateral tubal pregnancies. Hum Reprod 5:1025–1028, 1990.

33. Rizk B, Meagher S, Fisher AM. Severe ovarian hyperstimulation syndrome and cerebrovascular accidents. Hum Reprod 5:697–698, 1990.

34. Rizk B, Aboulghar M. Classification, pathophysiology and management of ovarian hyperstimulation syndrome. In Brinsden P, ed., A textbook of *in vitro* fertilization and assisted reproduction. Publishing, Carnforth, UK:Parthenon, 1999: Chapter 9; pp 131–155.

35. Rizk B, Smitz J. Ovarian hyperstimulation syndrome after superovulation for IVF and related procedures. Hum Reprod 7:320–327, 1992.

36. Rizk B, Aboulghar M. Modern management of ovarian hyperstimulation syndrome. Hum Reprod 6:1082–1087, 1991.

37. Egbase PE, Makhseed M, Al Sharhan M, *et al.* Timed unilateral ovarian follicular aspiration prior to administration of human chorionic gonadotropin for the prevention of severe ovarian hyperstimulation syndrome in *in vitro* fertilization: a prospective, randomized study. Hum Reprod 12:2603–2606, 1997.

38. Almeida OD Jr, Rizk B. Microlaparoscopic ovarian drilling under local anesthesia. Middle East Fertil Soc J 3:189–191, 1998.

MICROLAPAROSCOPY IN ASSISTED REPRODUCTIVE TECHNOLOGY

MOSTAFA I. ABUZEID, M.D., F.A.C.O.G., F.R.C.O.G.

Since the introduction of in vitro fertilization (IVF) for the treatment of tubal factor infertility, many advances in the field of assisted reproductive technology (ART) have been made. Initial success of IVF/embryo transfer was relatively low; however, results have improved over the last several years due to advances in culture technique, availability of knowledge, improved expertise by embryologists, and better understanding of ovulation induction by reproductive endocrinologists. Implantation rates remain relatively low, and every unit tries to improve its results in different ways.

Over the years, several units have reported higher pregnancy rates after tubal transfer of gametes, zygotes, or embryos (1,2). Tubal transfer requires additional surgery with the risk of further surgery, general anesthesia, and increased cost. Earlier attempts to simplify tubal transfer of gametes have proven to be fruitless. Some groups tried hysteroscopic gamete intrafallopian transfer (GIFT), but the results were disappointing (3). Other investigators tried to perform GIFT and zygote intrafallopian transfer (ZIFT) under ultrasound scan guidance; however the results were poor (4). It is believed that the trauma during transcervical cannulation of the fallopian tube is partially responsible for the reduced pregnancy rates compared to GIFT under general anesthesia. In this chapter I present our initial experience of GIFT and tubal embryo transfer (TET) using microlaparoscopy under local anesthesia with conscious sedation.

PATIENT SELECTION

The general principles that determine whether a patient is a suitable candidate for tubal transfer of gametes, zygotes, or embryos are the same

Microlaparoscopy, Edited by Oscar D. Almeida, Jr.
ISBN 0-471-34574-1   Copyright © 2000 by Wiley-Liss, Inc.

TABLE 11.1. INDICATIONS FOR TUBAL TRANSFER DURING ART
PROCEDURES

- Unexplained infertility
- Endometriosis
- Male factor infertility
- Ovulatory disorder
- Cervical factor
- History of difficult transfer
    Cervical stenosis
    Difficult angle of cervical canal
- Repeated failure after IVF/ET

whether the patient is having the procedure performed under general anesthesia or conscious sedation. Such principles include at least one healthy, patent fallopian tube as determined by a hysterosalpingogram or laparoscopy with chromotubation. The presence of fimbrial phimosis or peritubal adhesions are not contraindications for tubal transfer if these are associated with endometriosis only. Any history of pelvic inflammatory disease, previous ectopic pregnancy, or positive *Chlamydia trachomatis* antibody titer are contraindications for tubal transfer, because the risk of ectopic pregnancy is increased. Indications for tubal transfer during ART procedures are summarized in Table 11.1. Table 11.2 lists some of the advantages of tubal transfer over transuterine transfer. Contraindications for tubal transfer under conscious sedation are presented in Table 11.3.

Some factors may increase the likelihood of procedure failure. Patient weight is very important. Microlaparoscopic tubal transfer under local anesthesia with conscious sedation is not recommended in obese patients. The procedure is more likely to fail in patients with a low pain tolerance and those who were not properly informed of what to expect during the procedure. Table 11.4 illustrates the factors affecting patient tolerance under conscious sedation. If a large number of follicles develop and the ovaries are markedly enlarged, as in some patients with polycystic ovarian disease, it may be technically difficult to visualize the tubes under conscious sedation unless undesirable manipulation is done. Furthermore, if the ovaries

TABLE 11.2. ADVANTAGES OF TUBAL TRANSFER OVER TRANSUTERINE
TRANSFER

- A more physiologic environment for the developing embryos
- Embryos are presumed to reach the uterine cavity at the correct stage of endometrial development
- More acceptable to certain religions

TABLE 11.3. CONTRAINDICATIONS FOR TUBAL TRANSFER UNDER
CONSCIOUS SEDATION

- Underlying medical conditions
  - Cardiac
  - Pulmonary
  - CNS
- Obesity
- Previous abdominal surgery especially midline incisions
- History of peritonitis
- Allergy to local anesthetic

are adherent in the pouch of Douglas or the ovarian fossae, the procedure
may be technically difficult to perform. The same is true if peritubal adhesions or fimbrial phimosis are present. Allergy to local anesthetics is a
contraindication.

INSTRUMENTATION AND TECHNIQUE

During the preliminary phase of our work, all procedures were performed
in a traditional hospital operating room. After the initial 10 cases, all procedures have been done in a well-equipped office microlaparoscopy suite.
The facility must have adequate equipment, personnel, policies, and guidelines. Table 11.5 lists the equipment that must be in the procedure room.

Before surgery, all patients must fast for a minimum of 7 h. On arrival
to our center, informed written consent is obtained. An intravenous line is
placed and a preload of lactated Ringer's solution is administered before
the patient is transferred to the operating room. If oocyte retrieval followed
by GIFT is planned, then the patient is placed in the dorsal lithotomy
position. If ZIFT or TET is planned, then the patient is placed in the supine

TABLE 11.4. FACTORS AFFECTING PATIENT TOLERANCE UNDER
CONSCIOUS SEDATION

- Good communication with the patient
- Limited manipulation
- Gentle handling of organs
- Restricting the volume of the pneumoperitoneum
- Maintaining intraperitoneal pressure around 10 mm Hg
- Surgical experience to limit duration of surgery
- Patient sedation

TABLE 11.5. LIST OF EQUIPMENT THAT MUST BE AVAILABLE WHEN OFFICE
MICROLAPAROSCOPY IS PERFORMED

- ECG Monitor
- BP with 5-min sampling
- Pulseoximeter
- An O_2 supply (line or tank)
- Suction
- An Ambu bag and several masks of assorted sizes
- A selection of nasal/oral airways
- Crash cart

position. The bladder is catheterized and the patient is sterily prepared and draped. Oxygen is administrated via a nasal cannula at 3 L/min. An anesthesiologist or nurse anesthetist in our operating room monitors the patient's vital signs and other parameters, including continuous electrocardiogram, transcutaneous oxygen saturation readings, heart rate, respirations, and blood pressure.

Transvaginal ultrasound scan-guided retrieval of the oocytes under intravenous sedation and analgesia with midazolam and fentanyl is performed. The surgeon then regloves and starts the GIFT procedure. At that time, a bolus of 1 mg of midazolam and 50 μg of fentanyl citrate are given intravenously. If TET or ZIFT are to be performed, the above medications are given prior the local anesthesia. The subumbilical, paraumbilical, and suprapubic area two finger breadth above the symphysis pubis in the midline are infiltrated with 1% lidocaine with epinephrine 1:100,000 buffered with sodium bicarbonate (10:1 dilution). Initially, a 28-gauge needle is used to infiltrate the skin and subcutaneous tissue. This is followed by the use of a 22-gauge needle for infiltration of the deeper layers down to the peritoneum. Another area is infiltrated either to the right or left of the midline, half-way between the umbilicus and symphysis pubis.

A Veress needle and 2-mm trocar sheath are simultaneously introduced into the abdominal cavity. After removal of the Veress needle, a 2-mm microlaparoscope is introduced confirming the intraperitoneal position of the endoscope. At this time 1L of CO_2 is insufflated over one minute duration. Intra-abdominal pressure is maintained at 10 mmHg. The patient is placed in slight Trendelenburg's position. A 3-mm accessory trocar is placed in the midline suprapubic area. The patient is asked to perform the Valsalva maneuver to facilitate accessory trocar insertion in the face of limited pneumoperitoneum. The GIFT trocar and cannula are placed approximately 2 cm lateral to the midline, medial to the superficial epigastric artery on the side opposite to the tube to be cannulated. The sharp trocar is removed and the blunt trocar inserted.

The serosanguinous fluid that is usually present in the pelvic cavity following oocyte retrieval is removed with a 2-mm suction cannula attached to the vacuum apparatus. An atraumatic grasper placed through the suprapubic port is used to elevate the uterus gently to allow complete suction of the serosanguinous fluid from the pelvis. Using the atraumatic grasper, the antimesenteric end of the fimbria is elevated gently and the tube straightened and cannulated to a distance of 2 cm. The inner catheter is loaded with the gametes and passed through the outer catheter into the fallopian tube. The tip of the inner catheter is advanced 2 cm beyond that of the outer cannula before the transfer. The cannula and inner catheter are withdrawn slowly and examined by the embryologist for residual oocytes, zygotes, or embryos. The pneumoperitoneum is deflated as thoroughly as possible. After the removal of the trocars, the incision sites are approximated with Steri-strips. The patient is monitored postoperatively for 2 to 3 h before being discharged home.

Our preliminary results of microlaparoscopy and tubal transfer of gametes, zygotes, and embryos under local anesthesia with conscious sedation compare favorably with our own results and the results of other series using general anesthesia. The pregnancy and delivery rates are 44 and 41%, respectively, which are significantly higher than those of IVF/ET (32 and 25%, respectively). The 1995 delivery rates reported by the Society for Assisted Reproductive Technology registry, IVF/ET (22.5%) and GIFT (27%), were significantly lower than our delivery rate of 41% (5). There were no intraoperative or postoperative complications in our series. There was a high acceptance rate of 90%, and only 5% of patients had a poor acceptance rate. In 5% of patients, the procedure was canceled due to poor tolerance, and transuterine embryo transfer was performed instead.

Milki and Tazuke (6) compared CO_2 and air pneumoperitoneum for GIFT under local anesthesia with conscious sedation. They concluded that patient tolerance and pregnancy rates are similar for air and CO_2 pneumoperitoneum. Given the theoretical risk of air embolism and lack of detrimental effects of CO_2 on patient tolerance and the success rates, it seems prudent to use CO_2 in such settings. Milki and Tazuke (7) and Padilla et al. (8) used 5-mm laparoscopes to perform GIFT procedures in an office setting. The work by Milki and Tazuke (7) has demonstrated that office GIFT procedures under local anesthesia with conscious sedation can result in a high pregnancy and delivery rates of 43 and 38%, respectively. Furthermore, they reported high rates of patient acceptance (98%). There were no intraoperative or postoperative complications reported by either study (7,8).

The introduction of the 2-mm microlaparoscope has revolutionized the concept of office laparoscopy under local anesthesia with conscious sedation. We have used the 2-mm endoscope successfully to perform tubal transfer of gametes, zygotes, and embryos without any intraoperative or postoperative complications.

ADVANTAGES AND DISADVANTAGES OF OFFICE MICROLAPAROSCOPY

Office microlaparoscopy offers advantages for patients, practitioners, and managed care provider's which are detailed in Table 11.6.

There are some disadvantages of office microlaparoscopy for tubal transfer procedures. First, there are start-up costs and additional training requirements. At most ART programs, however, this may be minimal because many units have a facility, equipment, and personnel trained for oocyte retrieval procedures. In addition, the limited operative time, the limited field of view, the fragile equipment, and the fact that the patient is not paralyzed and asleep under general anesthesia make the procedure relatively difficult to perform. In cases where these limitations hinder tubal transfer, transcervical embryo transfer should be performed instead. The determining factors are patient selection and the skill of the surgeon. Both will limit the duration of surgery and increase the chances of successfully completing the procedure.

Potential complications are secondary to allergic reactions, overdose of local anesthetics, conscious sedation, or the actual surgical procedure. Injury to bowels and blood vessels during the introduction of 2-mm instruments is theoretically possible but rare. The possibility of injury to internal organs during introduction of 3-mm trocars and cannulas or GIFT trocars and cannulas can be eliminated by direct observation with a 2-mm microlaparoscope. Internal bleeding during the procedure can be avoided by the skill of the surgeon with gentle and minimal handling of tissues and limiting contact with the hyperstimulated ovaries, which can bleed easily. In addition, the procedure should not be performed if the ovaries are markedly enlarged or if the ovaries are fixed with adhesions deep in the pelvis. These situations require manipulation of organs and lifting the tube while the ovary is pulled down, which may lead to bleeding and make cannulation of the tube technically difficult. Risks secondary to local anesthesia could be eliminated by avoiding the use of excessive amounts of the local anesthetics and avoiding injecting the local anesthetic intravascularly.

TABLE 11.6. ADVANTAGES OF OFFICE MICROLAPAROSCOPY UNDER LOCAL ANESTHESIA WITH CONSCIOUS SEDATION

- Decreased scheduling delays
- Decreased preoperative delays
- Elimination of travel time and delays of practitioner
- Reduction in operative costs
- Decreased postoperative morbidity
- High rates of patient acceptance
- Fast rate of recovery

Complications secondary to medications used for conscious sedation should be reduced if one follows protocols and limits the dosage of the sedatives and by the presence of a skilled anesthetist or anesthesiologist.

SUMMARY

The potential advantages of performing ART under local anesthesia with conscious sedation are many. Tubal transfer of gametes, zygotes, and embryos can be performed by office microlaparoscopy under local anesthesia with conscious sedation. Procedures are well accepted by patients and provide scheduling flexibility, cost-effectiveness, patient safety, and a rapid recovery. The success rates are similar to those achieved during traditional laparoscopy under general anesthesia. Therefore, office microlaparoscopy for tubal transfer should be considered in favor of traditional laparoscopy under general anesthesia whenever tubal transfer is indicated.

REFERENCES

1. David L, Mashiach S, Dor J, Levron J, and Farhi J. Zygote intrafallopian transfer may improve pregnancy rate in patients with repeated failure of implantation. Fertil Steril 69:26–30, 1998.

2. Van Voorhis BJ, Chestnut DH, Syrop CH, et al. Tubal versus uterine transfer of cryopreserved embryos: a prospective randomized trial. Fertil Steril 63:578–583, 1995.

3. Bulmaceda JP, Manzur A. Current status of GIFT. Contemp Obstet Gynecol 12:59–71, 1993.

4. Hurst BS, Tucker KE, Guadagnolis A, et al. Transcervical gamete and zygote intrafallopian transfer: does it enhance pregnancy rates in an assisted reproduction program? J Reprod Med 41:867–870, 1996.

5. Society for Assisted Reproductive Technology and the American Society for Reproductive Medicine. Assisted reproductive technology in the United States and Canada: 1995 results generated from the American Society for Reproductive Medicine/Society for Assisted Reproductive Technology Registry. Fertil Steril 69:389–398, 1998.

6. Milki AA, Tazuke SL. Comparison of carbon dioxide and air pneumoperitoneum for gamete intrafallopian transfer under conscious sedation and local anesthesia. Fertil Steril 69:552–554, 1998.

7. Milki AA, Tazuke SL. Office laparoscopy under local anesthesia for gamete intrafallopian transfer: technique and tolerance. Fertil Steril 68:128–132, 1997.

8. Padilla SL, Dugan K, Maruschak V, et al. Laparoscopically assisted gamete intrafallopian transfer with local anesthesia and intravenous sedation. Fertil Steril 66:404–407, 1996.

MICROLAPAROSCOPIC OVARIAN DRILLING IN THE SURGICAL MANAGEMENT OF POLYCYSTIC OVARIAN SYNDROME

OSCAR D. ALMEIDA, JR., M.D., F.A.C.O.G., F.A.C.S., and
BOTROS RIZK, M.D., M.A., M.R.C.O.G., F.R.C.S.(C.),
H.C.L.D., F.A.C.O.G., F.A.C.S.

The treatment of polycystic ovarian syndrome continues to evolve. Today clomiphene citrate is the first line of treatment for anovulation. Unfortunately, 25% of anovulatory women do not respond to clomiphene and only 40 to 50% will conceive (1, 2). Women with PCOS who are resistant to medical therapy, those for whom medical therapy may be cost-prohibitive, and those who have concerns about multiple gestation may benefit from surgical treatment. Furthermore, it has been observed that the risk of miscarriage in pregnancies after laparoscopic electrosurgery is significantly lower than that after ovulation induction (3).

Many changes have taken place in the surgical management of polycystic ovarian syndrome since 1935 when Stein and Leventhal (4) first reported performing bilateral ovarian wedge resections via laparotomy on seven patients. They resected from one-half to three-fourths of each ovary. The patients were discharged from the hospital between the 9th and 13th postoperative day. Menstruation occurred on the 3rd to 5th postoperative day and monthly thereafter in all seven patients. Two of the patients were able to conceive.

Ovarian wedge resection is associated with a high incidence of periadnexal adhesions, which may jeopardize fertility (5). In 1984, Gjönnaess (6) introduced the laparoscopic method of ovarian cauterization. A total of 92% of

Microlaparoscopy, Edited by Oscar D. Almeida, Jr.
ISBN 0-471-34574-1   Copyright © 2000 by Wiley-Liss, Inc.

the 62 patients in his initial study ovulated and 24 of 35 who were involuntarily sterile achieved pregnancy. Gjönnaess's technique produces similar positive results to bilateral ovarian resection, either by laparoscopy or laparotomy, but is more minimally invasive with less surgical trauma. These remarkable results demonstrated that the more surgically invasive method of ovarian wedge resection could be substituted for a less invasive procedure.

A novel variation of an established technique for the surgical management of PCOS is showing great promise (7). In 1998, we reported the first case of microlaparoscopic ovarian drilling under local anesthesia. Since that initial case, many more cases have been performed with equal success.

TECHNIQUE

After our conscious sedation protocol (atropine 0.2 mg, ondansetron hydrochloride 4 mg, midazolam hydrochloride 2 mg, and fentanyl citrate 250 µg titrated to effect), a paracervical block is administered (1% lidocaine with epinephrine 1:100,000, 10 mL buffered with sodium bicarbonate 8.4% concentration 10:1 dilution) and a uterine manipulator is placed in utero (8). After administering a periumbilical block, a 2-mm cannula and Veress needle are inserted and the abdomen is insufflated with 3 L carbon dioxide. Although we use less insufflation (usually 1.5 L) for all other cases, the additional pneumoperitoneum is necessary to isolate the adnexae in these frequently obese patients. Once the microlaparoscope is inserted, two additional anesthetic blocks are placed over the right and left suprapubic regions, and a 2-mm trocar is inserted at each site into the pelvic cavity.

After applying 1% plain lidocaine over each ovarian cortex several times to allow absorption of the local anesthetic, the utero-ovarian ligament is grasped with a 2-mm grasper for stabilization of the ovary (Fig. 12.1).

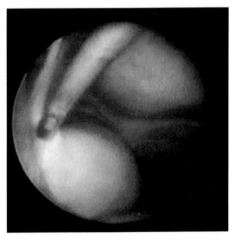

FIGURE 12.1. Stabilization of the ovary is achieved by grasping the utero-ovarian ligament.

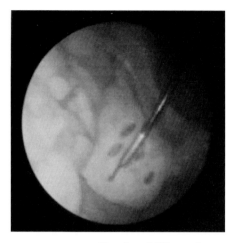

FIGURE 12.2. Ovarian drilling using
the 2-mm cautery scissors.

With the ovary held away from the bowel and other vital structures, a minimum of 10 holes penetrating the cortex of the ovary, 3 to 4-mm in diameter
and approximately 5-mm deep are burned over the surface of the ovary using 2-mm cautery scissors at a power setting of 30 W monopolar pinpoint
coagulation (Figs. 12.2 and 12.3). A similar procedure is then employed on
the contralateral ovary.

The sites of ovarian drilling are usually hemostatic. Sutures are not
required on the ovary or the skin. We have encountered no technical limitations for this procedure other than performing operative microlaparoscopy
under local anesthesia in obese patients. The duration of the procedures
from the first incision to removal of the trocars at the conclusion has been
approximately 25 min. All women have remained comfortable and con-
versed with us during their procedures.

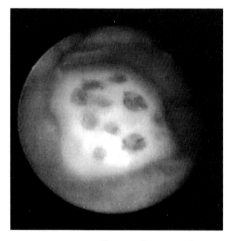

FIGURE 12-3. Ovary after microlaparoscopic ovarian drilling.

After monitoring the patients for 1 h postoperatively in the recovery room, patients are discharged home on oral Lortab 7.5 mg, 1 to 2 every 4 h as needed for pain. All patients have returned to their usual activities within 1 week of their surgery.

SUMMARY

Microlaparoscopic ovarian drilling presents tremendous advantages over traditional methods done with larger instrumentation and under general anesthesia. Using our technique, the procedures are performed in a very minimally invasive manner and produce less surgical trauma, thus decreasing the risk of adhesion formation. The preliminary results from our ongoing series appear to be similar to those reported in the literature with macrolaparoscopy under general anesthesia in regard to return of menses and pregnancy rate. With cauterization, only a small area of the ovarian cortex and subcortical tissue is destroyed compared to at least 50% of the ovary during wedge resection. Furthermore, the sites of ovarian drilling do not require suturing and the risk of hemorrhage is decreased. This technique should be considered whenever medical therapy is an undesirable option.

REFERENCES

1. Garcia J, Jones GS, Wentz AC. The use of clomiphene citrate. Gertil Steril 28:707–717, 1977.
2. Gorlitzky GA, Kase NG, Speroff L. Ovulation and pregnancy rates with clomiphene citrate. Obstet Gynecol 51:265–269, 1978.
3. Gadir AA, Khatim MS, Mowafi RS. Ovarian electrocautery versus HMG and pure FSH therapy in the treatment of patients with PCOS. Clin Endocrinol 33:582–592, 1990.
4. Stein IF, Leventhal ML. Amenorrhea associated with bilateral polycystic ovaries. Am J Obstet Gynecol 29:181–191, 1935.
5. Naether OGJ. Significant reduction of adnexal adhesions following laparoscopi electrocautery of the ovarian surface by lavage and artificial ascites. Gynaecol Endosc 4:17–19, 1995.
6. Gjönnaess H. Polycystic ovarian syndrome treated by ovarian electrocautery through the laparoscope. Fertil Steril 41:20–25, 1984.
7. Almeida OD Jr, Rizk B. Microlaparoscopic ovarian drilling under local anesthesia. Middle East Fertil Soc J. 3:189–191, 1998.
8. Almeida OD Jr, Val-Gallas JM, Browning JL. A protocol for conscious sedation in microlaparoscopy. J Am Assoc Gynecol Laparosc 4:591–594, 1997.

CREDENTIALING FOR MICROLAPAROSCOPY AND NEGOTIATING CONTRACTS FOR OFFICE MICROLAPAROSCOPY

OSCAR D. ALMEIDA, JR., M.D., F.A.C.O.G., F.A.C.S.

CREDENTIALING

Although as of this writing there are no standardized guidelines specifically relating to *microlaparoscopy*, through our 2-day course Advanced Diagnostic and Operative Microlaparoscopy under Local Anesthesia, which includes a didactic course and hands-on, supervised laboratory experience using live porcine models, we have served as a credentialing instrument throughout the country for many gynecology departments that wish to embark on this new technology (call 334–639–1847 for more information). Physicians interested in performing microlaparoscopy—whether in the hospital, outpatient ambulatory surgery center, or their own office microlaparoscopy suite—are encouraged to attend one of our courses or another similar course.

It is predicted that in the near future, gynecologists are going to require a greater fund of knowledge in the area of conscious sedation. Many procedures once done only in the traditional hospital operating room are now being performed in the physician's office. Managed care organizations are currently evaluating a more widespread use of diagnostic and operative laparoscopy without the use of general anesthesia in selected patients.

Most gynecologists are unfamiliar with the safe administration of intravenous conscious sedation. Our protocol for conscious sedation in microlaparoscopy provides useful guidelines (1). It is a totally new experience to perform laparoscopic surgery on an awake patient and goes beyond the

Microlaparoscopy, Edited by Oscar D. Almeida, Jr.
ISBN 0-471-34574-1   Copyright © 2000 by Wiley-Liss, Inc.

scope of training for most gynecologists. The new 2-mm microinstrumentation requires a great skill level owing to fragility of the instruments. In addition, because of their size, if used inappropriatelly they may cause more bleeding. Therefore, microlaparoscopy requires advanced training even for the experienced laparoscopist.

Most hospital gynecology departments have specific laparoscopic training requirements that appear to be uniformly employed to perform advanced laparoscopic surgery.

These include the following:

1. The applicant is board eligible or certified by the American Board of Obstetrics and Gynecology.

2. The applicant must be a member in good standing in their respective department of obstetrics and gynecology where the procedures are to be performed.

3. The applicant must be previously credentialed in diagnostic and operative laparoscopy. This credentialing requires documentation of satisfactory training in this area with a letter of certification of competence either during residency training or CME Continuing Medical Education approved didactic and hands on learning followed by a preceptorship. The number of cases and hours of preceptorship are determined by each individual department.

The procedures that can be performed by gynecologists either via laparoscopy or laparotomy vary among hospitals. Unfortunately, some hospitals and ambulatory surgery centers limit which procedures can be performed even by competent gynecologic surgeons owing to turf battles between the gynecologists and general surgeons. A prime example is the laparoscopic appendectomy, which is technically easy to perform and should be seriously considered in women who suffer from chronic pelvic pain.

NEGOTIATING CONTRACTS

The purpose of this section is to provide the physician who wishes to embark on performing office microlaparoscopy with some general information regarding contracts and to relate my experience in dealing with managed care organizations in this regard. First, it should be mentioned that at this time there is no current procedural terminology (CPT) code specifically designated for office microlaparoscopy. Therefore, negotiations must be conducted on a case-by-case situation, more precisely on a practice-by-practice scenario.

To be worthwhile, (both professionally and financially) setting up an office microlaparoscopy suite cannot cause the practice to lose money. Many insurance carriers will pay you your usual customary professional fee for doing a given procedure in the office, such as microlaparoscopic lysis of adhesions, however, because at this time few carriers will reimburse you for a facility fee, your customary surgeon's fees are not enough to cover the expenses incurred when performing the procedure in the office. When you include equipment use, supplies, and additional staff, you end up either losing money or barely breaking even, which makes the endeavor not worthwhile.

The approach that we have taken in our practice is to demonstrate to the third-party payers that the reimbursement for office microlaparoscopic procedures is actually a win-win situation for all parties involved. The patient wins because she has her procedure performed in a minimally invasive fashion in a facility that she is familiar with (i.e., her doctor's office versus a hospital operating room). The managed care organization/insurance carrier comes out ahead because when it compares costs head to head between the same procedure being done in the office versus the hospital operating room, the office procedure results in a cost savings of thousands of dollars. One study reported that billed charges were reduced up to 80% when the laparoscopic procedure was performed in the office laparoscopy suite (2). Because we administer our own intravenous conscious sedation by our trained physician/nursing ACLS-certified staff, there is no anesthesiologist fee that the insurance carrier has to pay. Owing to the increased effort in the setup of the office microlaparoscopy suite, increased skill level necessary to perform microlaparoscopy and to administer conscious sedation safely, the physicians are financially compensated at a higher level than if the procedures were performed in the hospital operating room.

What this has translated to in our practice is the following. We bill for our customary surgeon's and assistant surgeon's fees for the given procedure in addition to a negotiated "facility fee." The way to calculate your facility fee varies and depends on several factors. First, determine the cost of your surgical supplies, including all drugs used for the procedure. Evaluate what type of effort is necessary to prepare the suite for surgery (e.g., housekeeping needs, including special cleaning procedures). Take into account what special equipment has been purchased to perform these procedures and come up with a fair dollar amount for its use during a procedure. Finally, consider any additional training required by the physicians, nurses, and ancillary staff to function as a surgical team. This includes not only courses on microlaparoscopic technique but the administration of conscious sedation and ACLS certification of the physicians and registered nurse. The facility fee plus the surgeon's and assistant surgeon's customary surgical fee, once expenses are subtracted, should provide a markedly higher revenue for the physicians, making their efforts worthwhile. Therefore, it is also a win-win situation for the physicians.

Several criteria are usually required (appropriately so) by the managed care organizations/insurance carriers before they will contract you to provide microlaparoscopy services in your office. First, the facility must be specially adapted to perform such functions safely and effectively. The microlaparoscopy suite must be set up the same as you would have in a traditional hospital operating room with the exception of general anesthesia. Emergency equipment such as monitors (heart rate, ECG, respirations, pulseoximeter, and blood pressure), crash cart (containing emergency medications and reversal agents), defibrillator, and oxygen supply must be available. The physicians must show documentation of training in microlaparoscopy and the administration of conscious sedation. The physicians and registered nurse must show documentation of being currently ACLS certified. Finally, an emergency plan containing details of action, emergency telephone numbers, and protocols for patient transport and hospital admission should be located in the operating room. An on-site visit by the managed care organization/insurance carrier will be conducted to document that the above criteria have been met.

REFERENCES

1. Almeida OD Jr, Val-Gallas JM, Browning JL. A protocol for conscious sedation in microlaparoscopy. J Am Assoc Gynecol Laparosc 4:591–594, 1977.
2. Palter SF, Olive DL. Office microlaparoscopy under local anesthesia for chronic pelvic pain. J Am Assoc Gynecol Laparosc 3:359–364, 1996.

ATLAS

The following photographs were chosen to illustrate the visual signs of normal and abnormal findings during diagnostic and operative microlaparoscopic procedures. With the expanding field of microlaparoscopy, previously unpublished photographs such as those obtained during the first microlaparoscopic tubal anastomosis under local anesthesia with conscious sedation are presented.

All photographs were taken by Oscar D. Almeida, Jr., M.D., F.A.C.O.G., F.A.C.S., using a 2-mm, 50,000-pixel fiberoptic microlaparoscope. Anyone who has performed microlaparoscopy using this 2-mm microlaparoscope has experienced the excellent clarity of view, comparable to a traditional rod lens laparoscope, during the procedures.

Regardless of the videotape or laparoscopic camera used, the image noted during the live procedure is always of higher quality and resolution than that noted when the videotape is reviewed. In obtaining the pictures for this atlas, three steps were required, which minimally compromised picture resolution in the process. From the videos obtained during actual cases, the videotapes were paused at the desired picture frames. The pictures were then copied with the use of a computer and the image placed on a floppy disk. The disk was then sent to the printers for subsequent printing. Most pictures are self-explanatory with their captions; additional comments are provided when needed. It is hoped that these pictures will further stimulate the laparoscopic surgeon to employ these minimally invasive techniques.

Microlaparoscopy, Edited by Oscar D. Almeida, Jr.
ISBN 0-471-34574-1   Copyright © 2000 by Wiley-Liss, Inc.

NORMAL ANATOMY

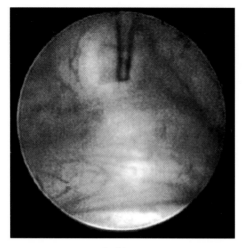

FIGURE A.1. Bladder peritoneum and upper portion of the uterus.

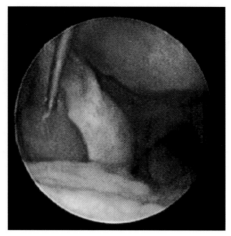

FIGURE A.2. Adnexa.

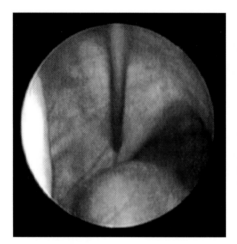

FIGURE A.3. Uterosacral ligament.

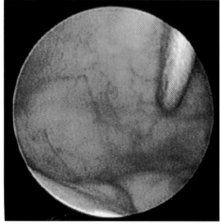

FIGURE A.4. Posterior cul-de-sac (pouch of Douglas).

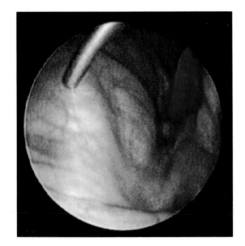

FIGURE A.5. Pelvic side wall.

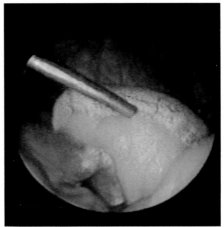

FIGURE A.6. Appendix.

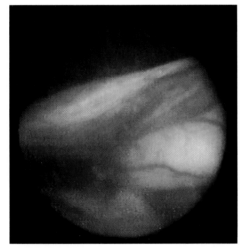

FIGURE A.7. Liver.

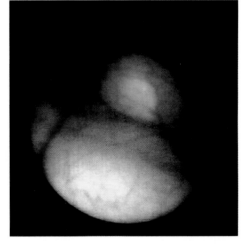

FIGURE A.8. Gallbladder.

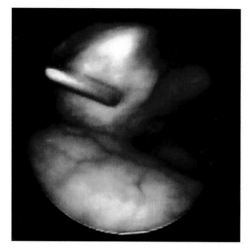

FIGURE A.9. Ovary and adjacent small bowel.

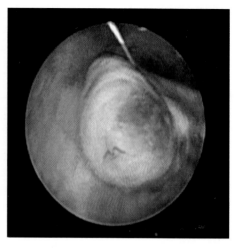

FIGURE A.10. Unruptured ovarian follicle.

ABNORMAL ANATOMY AND DIAGNOSTIC AND OPERATIVE PROCEDURES

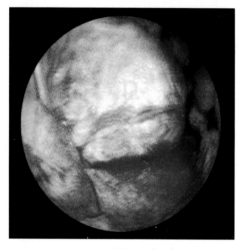

FIGURE A.11. Enlarged hemorrhagic ovarian cyst. Note the hypervascularity and hemorrhage.

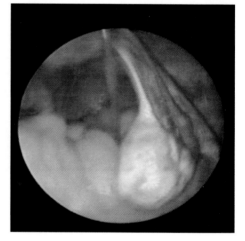

FIGURE A.12. Adnexa with a polycystic ovary.

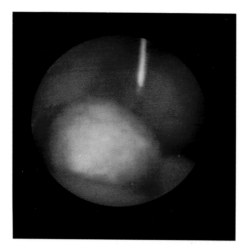

FIGURE A.13. Polycystic ovary.

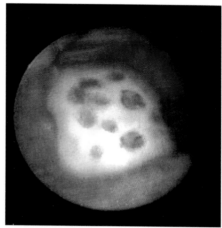

FIGURE A.14. Ovary after microlaparoscopic ovarian drilling. Multiple sites of fulguration are noted on the ovarian cortex.

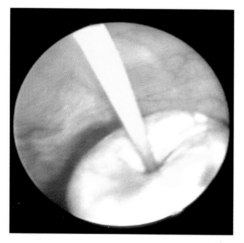

FIGURE A.15. Drainage of ovarian cyst. Partial collapse of the cyst wall after aspiration of fluid.

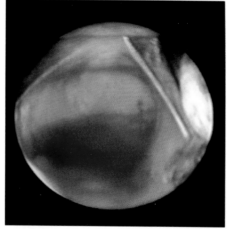

FIGURE A.16. Posterior cul-de-sac (pouch of Douglas) containing fluid from a rupture ovarian cyst. Note the amount of fluid still remaining after aspiration of 90 mL from an apparent ruptured ovarian cyst.

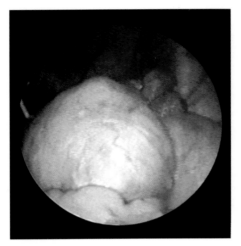

FIGURE A.17. Enlarged simple ovarian cyst. This cyst was approximately 8 cm in diameter and produced pain due to its size. Initial aspiration of fluid before excision of the cyst wall yielded 130 mL of fluid.

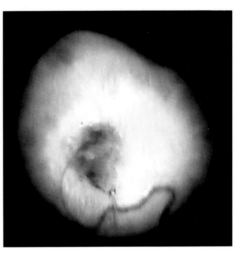

FIGURE A.18. Dermoid cyst (cystic teratoma) with hair.

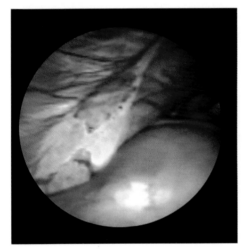

FIGURE A.19. Classical "black" endometriosis lesion. Note the varying degrees of fibrosis and dark pigmentation. These are often considered to be burned out lesions and are noted to be the least painful during conscious pain mapping.

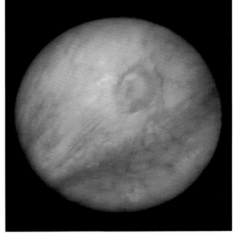

FIGURE A.20. Classical "powder-burn" endometriosis lesion.

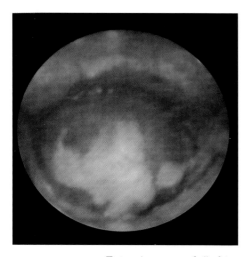

FIGURE A.21. Extensive serosal "white endometriosis" of the uterus. Biopsy of this tissue revealed endometriosis.

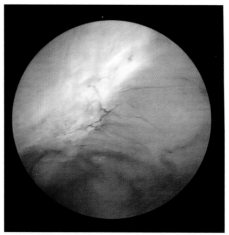

FIGURE A.22. Atypical "white endometriosis" presenting on the pelvic side wall. These white lesions are noted when there is an absence of hemorrhage and probably represent early stages of development before vascularization.

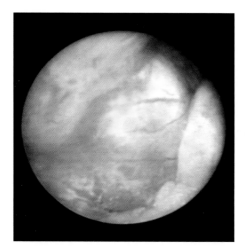

FIGURE A.23. Typical and atypical endometriosis of the posterior cul-de-sac (pouch of Douglas). Note both the fibrosis and the pigmentation as well as the "white" lesions.

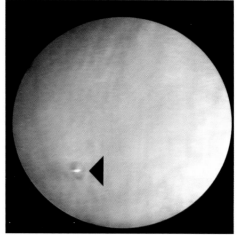

FIGURE A.24. Atypical vesicular implant. These small, clear lesions may occur as single or multiple lesions. The vesicles result from fluid accumulation between the surface of the endometriotic implant and the overlying peritoneum. These early vesicular implants are frequently painful to probing during conscious pain mapping.

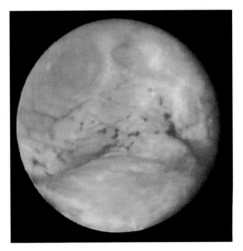

FIGURE A.25. Endometriosis over the bladder peritoneum. Atypical endometriosis presenting as hypervascularity and "red" lesions.

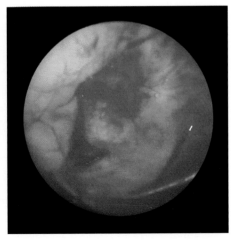

FIGURE A.26. Atypical red "endometriosis" of the side wall. This picture reveals extensive hemorrhage and hypervascularity. These active lesions have been noted to be the most painful endometriotic lesions during conscious pain mapping.

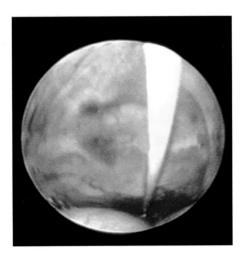

FIGURE A.27. Atypical endometriosis of the posterior cul-de-sac (pouch of Douglas). Red hemorrhagic and white avascular lesions are noted.

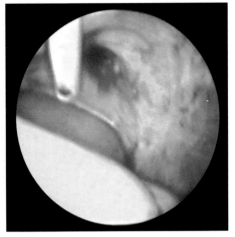

FIGURE A.28. Hemorrhagic peritoneal pocket in the posterior cul-de-sac (Pouch of Douglas). Note the atypical red hemorrhagic implants and the white avascular lesions.

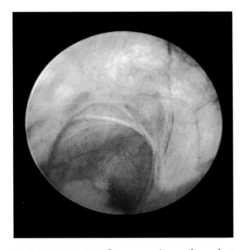

FIGURE A.29. Large peritoneal pocket in the posterior cul-de-sac (pouch of Douglas). Note the atypical white endometriosis above the endometriosis crypt.

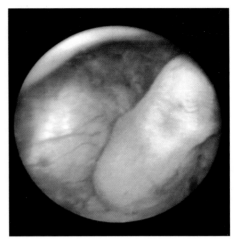

FIGURE A.30. Hydrosalpinx (pyosalpinx). Note the typical "powder-burn" endometriosis implants in the cul-de-sac.

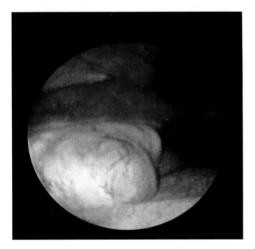

FIGURE A.31. Endometrioma.

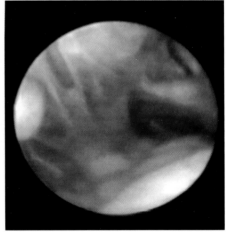

FIGURE A.32. Obliteration of the cul-de-sac in stage IV endometriosis.

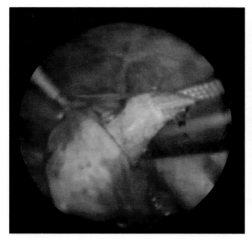

FIGURE   A.33. Endosalpingiosis of the ovary.

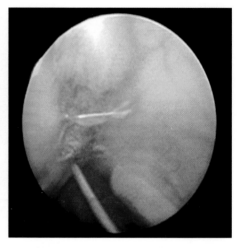

FIGURE A.34. White scarification of the pelvic side wall.

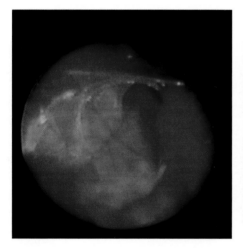

FIGURE A.35. Adnexal adhesions.

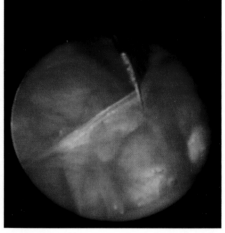

FIGURE A.36. Microlaparoscopic lysis of peritubal adhesions.

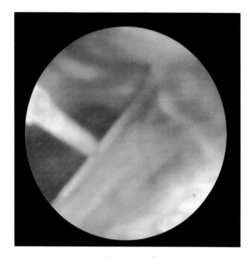

FIGURE A.37. Lysis of vascular adhesions.

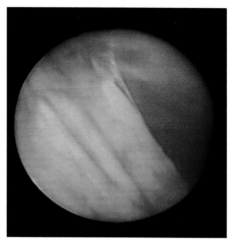

FIGURE A.38. Abdominal wall omental adhesions after a cholecystectomy.

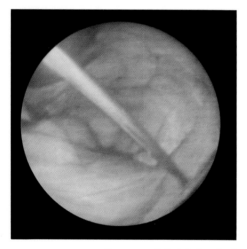

FIGURE A.39. Severe pelvic/abdominal adhesions distorting anatomy.

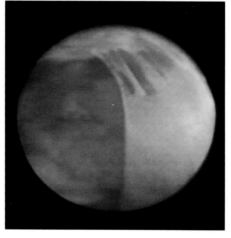

FIGURE A.40. Small bowel adherent to the anterior abdominal wall.

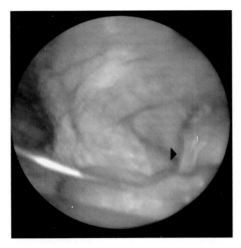

FIGURE A.41. Small bowel to bowel adhesions (*arrow*).

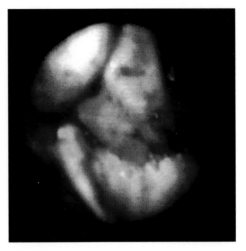

FIGURE A.42. Crohn's disease (regional enteritis).

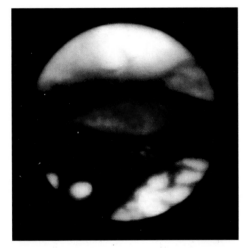

FIGURE A.43. Hemoperitoneum resulting from a ruptured ectopic pregnancy.

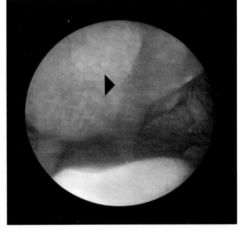

FIGURE A.44. Inclusion cyst (*arrow*) of the uterus secondary to a chronic inflammatory response.

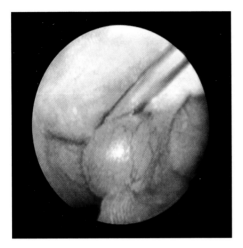

FIGURE A.45. Paratubal cyst (para-mesonephric duct remnant).

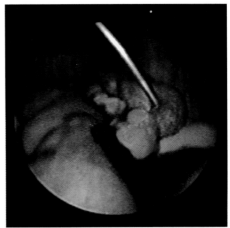

FIGURE A.46. Assessment of tubal patency with indigo carmine dye.

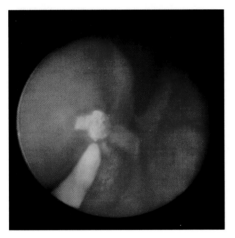

FIGURE A.47. Hulka clip method of tubal sterilization.

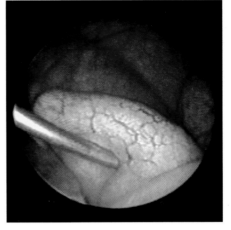

FIGURE A.48. Abnormal appendix with proximal dilatation secondary to a fecalith.

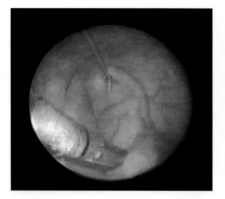

FIGURE A.49. Microlaparoscopic appendectomy using a 2-mm grasper and linear stapling device.

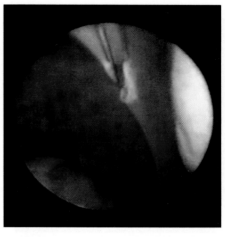

FIGURE A.50. Microlaparoscopic LUNA.

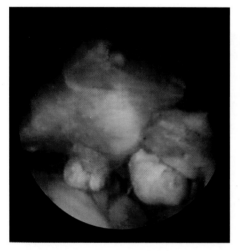

FIGURE A.51. Uterine fibroids.

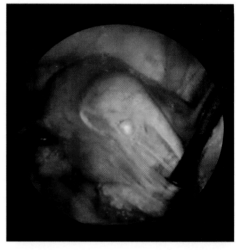

FIGURE A.52. Chronic pelvic inflammatory disease. Note the extensive adnexal adhesions.

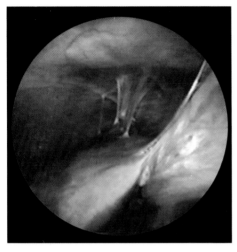

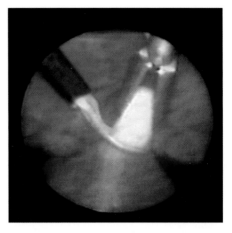

FIGURE A.53. Fitz-Hugh-Curtis syndrome.

FIGURE A.54. Microlaparoscopic myomectomy.

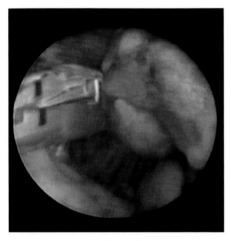

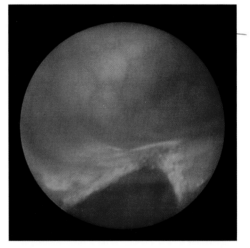

FIGURE A.55. Microlaparoscopic assisted vaginal hysterectomy using a linear stapling device.

FIGURE A.56. Staple lines (*at bottom*) from linear stapling device.

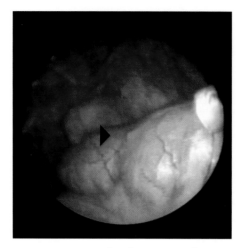

FIGURE A.57. Small trocar perforation of the small bowel bowel. Note the bowel contents leaking from the site of perforation (*arrow*) before irrigation.

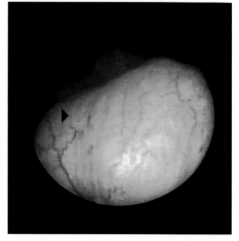

FIGURE A.58. Site of small bowel perforation (*arrow*) after irrigation with saline. Note that no further leakage of bowel contents or active hemorrhage is noted at the site of injury. Bowel injuries resulting from 2-mm trocars or Veress needles can be managed conservatively without suturing of the bowel, provided that the site does not leak any further bowel contents and is hemostatic.

MICROLAPAROSCOPIC TUBAL ANASTOMOSIS UNDER LOCAL ANESTHESIA

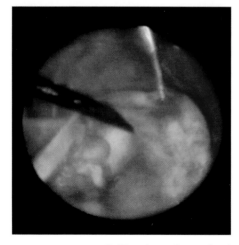

FIGURE A.59. Infiltration of proximal tube segment with pitressin solution to enhance hemostasis.

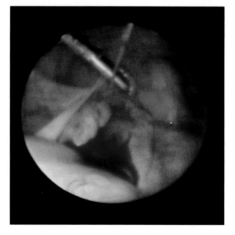

FIGURE A.60. Infiltration of distal tube segment with pitressin solution.

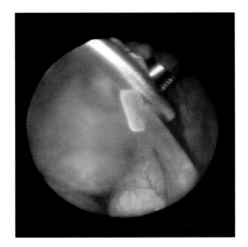

FIGURE A.61. Cutting proximal tube segment.

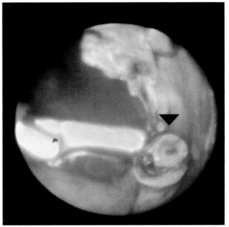

FIGURE A.62. Cross-section view of cut distal tube segment (*arrow*) with patent lumen.

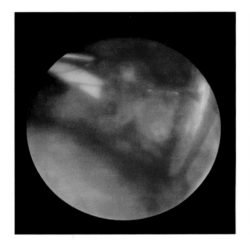

FIGURE A.63. Insertion of stent in fallopian tube lumen.

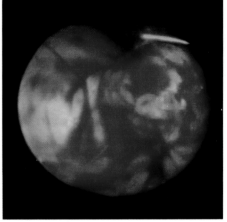

FIGURE A.64. Approximation of tube segments partially sutured.

INDEX